Evidence-based health communication

Evidence-based health communication

Brian Brown
Paul Crawford
Ronald Carter

 Open University Press

Open University Press
McGraw-Hill Education
McGraw-Hill House
Shoppenhangers Road
Maidenhead
Berkshire
England
SL6 2QL

email: enquiries@openup.co.uk
world wide web: www.openup.co.uk

and Two Penn Plaza, New York, NY 10121–2289, USA

First published 2006

Copyright © Brian Brown, Paul Crawford and Ronald Carter 2006

A catalogue record of this book is available from the British Library

ISBN–10: 0 335 21995 0 (pb) 0 335 21996 9 (hb)
ISBN–13: 978 0 335 21995 7 (pb) 978 0 335 21996 4 (hb)

Library of Congress Cataloguing-in-Publication Data
CIP data applied for

Typeset by YHT Ltd, London
Printed in Poland by OZ Graf. S.A.
www.polskabook.pl

The **McGraw·Hill** Companies

Acknowledgements

This volume would not have been possible without the support, discussion and generous sharing of ideas between colleagues that has taken place at the Nottingham Heath Language Research Group. We would particularly like to thank Kevin Harvey, Alison Pilnick, Nicola Gray, Chris Candlin and Srikant Sarangi. But thanks must also go to many others – practitioners, clients, research participants, friends and families who have shared their experiences with us and have enabled our thinking to develop, as well as a supportive team at Open University Press who helped bring the project to fruition. Any errors are, of course, our own.

Contents

1 Theories of health communication and theories of society

Why communication? Why theory?

There are a variety of ways in which we might think about what happens in the myriad encounters of health care and how these might be linked to what happens in the societies within which they are embedded. For health care encounters will inevitably be influenced and shaped by a wide range of social, cultural, political and economic factors. In this opening chapter we will consider how the process of health care communication might be conceptualized to take this into account. After all, it is difficult to leave one's whole life history and socio-economic position outside the consulting room door, whether one is a client or a professional. Equally, many thinkers have been trying to make sense of how social inequalities are manifest in the health care encounter itself.

Health care professionals are often relatively privileged compared with their clients. Most societies show a distinct pattern of health inequality. The less well off a person is, the more likely they will be to suffer a whole variety of illnesses. Indeed, there are suggestions that some indicators of health such as infant mortality and life expectancy are showing a widening gap between rich and poor in the UK (Department of Health 2005a; Shaw et al. 2005). So from the outset, the social and economic context has a bearing on health care activity. There may be other broader social factors at work. People may differ markedly in terms of their access to knowledge, language and 'social capital' in relation to health care (Edmondson 2003). An individual's social and cultural capital can make a substantial difference to how accessible health services are, and how user-friendly they find them to be. The terms 'social capital' and 'cultural capital' refer to resources based on group membership, relationships, networks of influence and social support. They relate to advantages a person might have, linked to their position in networks of social relationships, and might also reflect knowledge, skill, education, and other advantages which give certain people a higher status in society, and possibly higher expectations.

Social factors, then, have an important bearing on health. As we shall see in this volume, they influence health care encounters too. In this first chapter we will begin the task of picking out some of the theories that have been used to make sense of health, and suggest some others which are perhaps less familiar to scholars of health care but which we feel have some potential to offer insights into how one can make sense of the sometimes problematic relationship between what happens in the health care encounter and the wider world.

Originally, in the 1950s and 1960s when the discipline of medical sociology was finding its feet in American universities, social scientists visited hospital settings, with a view to describing, explaining and theorizing what they saw. At that time in

American social science a view of social life called 'functionalism' was very popular such that sickness, disease and death were often seen in terms of their functions within a broader social structure. Since then, the study of health care has turned out to be fertile soil for researchers and theorists to grow illustrious careers and deploy a whole variety of perspectives. Thus, as well as traditional social theory perspectives such as functionalism and Marxism, we can see newer and sometimes more critical perspectives such as feminism, social constructionism, postmodernism and even branches of literary theory creating significant inroads into the field.

While these developments were going on in social science, the health professions themselves were becoming more interested in the role of communication in their daily work. This was most pronounced in nursing, which has recently seen the 50th anniversary of Hildegard Peplau's landmark volume *Interpersonal Relations in Nursing* (1952). Since then, there have been many attempts to characterize the role of communication, storytelling and textual practice in the discipline of nursing (Crawford et al 1998, Frid et al. 2000; Taylor 2003; Nelson and McGillion 2004). These developments have been echoed in other disciplines such as medicine (Das Gupta 2003) with a growing recognition that the study of language, communication and literature

> opens up a wealth of experience and knowledge, as well as offering vital understandings of the narrative nature of human lives. A knowledge of the nature of narrative, and the way we understand our lives narratively can be vital for effective communication and understanding of patients' situations.
> (Bolton 2005: 171)

Other disciplines have climbed aboard this bandwagon, including occupational therapy (Goldstein et al. 2004) and dentistry (Schouten et al. 2003) but it is nursing that has pioneered this recent interest in the English-speaking world.

However, reading the literature and coming across extended reflective narratives, disquisitions on meaning and considerations of communicative practice in the learned journals of a health care discipline, and in professional trainings, might be misleading. In the half-century since Peplau (1952) famously described nursing as an interpersonal process, the size of caseloads and lists in many care settings means that in practice Peplau's interpersonal legacy is sometimes in danger of seeming like a quaint carry-over from a bygone age. As we shall show, some of the original edicts of good communication practice originated in specialist counselling practices – a further offshoot of Peplau's (1964) pioneering work which often assumed a luxury of time and space which many health settings cannot muster. Nowadays, even in psychotherapy and counselling, the trend towards brevity, and the popularity of solution-focused therapies, has noticeably squeezed the spaces available for clients to unfold their narratives.

Such trends suggest that brief communications are likely to play an increasing role in health care in the future. This is a topic which we shall delve into in Chapter 10, but for now it is important to bear in mind that there may seldom be time in contemporary health care practice for the extended interventions written about in accounts of psychotherapy or story sharing. Perhaps instead we need to explore the usefulness of quick, generic and pragmatic communication along an axis of skilled ordinariness. As Burnard (2003: 682) puts it, when talking about mental health nurses, they 'may be remembered as much for their friendliness and ordinariness as for their counselling skills. Ordinary chat might be as important as therapeutic conversation'. Therefore, brevity and ordinariness have an important role to play. This would appear to be a fairly straightforward, achievable goal. Yet this may not be the case, even when we want to bring about such change. As contemporary popular idiom has it: 'It's not rocket science'.

Another reason why it is useful to consider theories of communication in relation to theories of society and social change is that we study communication because very often we want to change it. Improved communication is believed to enhance a whole variety of outcomes from lower levels of depression and anxiety (Davies 2000) to lower rates of stillbirths and infant deaths (Rowe et al. 2001). It is often difficult in practice to get people to improve their communicative activities. The practitioners may all be 'perfectly nice people', often superbly capable of making their own friends and family members feel good, even from a very brief interaction. Yet in Kasper's (1997: 2) words, they 'don't always use what they know' in professional contexts. In a sense it is as difficult to change communication patterns in health care as it is to change society itself.

Designing in good practice: why we don't all do the right thing

Another set of important lessons in the development of learning about communication for health professionals comes from the design professions such as ergonomics and engineering. Here the process of getting people to adopt innovative technologies has been a problem for some time. In health care a number of commentators have lamented how the basic problem of communication between client and professional remains despite all the training, professional development and consultation protocols that have proliferated in the last 20 years. Trying to get people to communicate differently is rather like trying to get them to adopt technologies, or undertake innovative agriculture strategies or hygiene practices. Students of innovation in other disciplines talk of the contrast between 'revolution' and 'legacy' (Crabtree 2003). Innovators and educators often seek to revolutionize practice with new techniques and technologies, but as Crabtree argues, the more successful innovations seek to build on a legacy of practice.

Maybe one of the reasons why many innovations in health care designed to enhance communication have had less than encouraging results is that they have not paid enough attention to what is already there. The legacy of existing practice is often deeply ingrained and serves important social functions. Perhaps one way of enhancing the success of new initiatives is not to ignore the existing organized practices found in health care, but to build upon them (Mitchell 2000). While there have been revolutions in the way human beings have seen themselves (Brown et al. 2003) there are many curious continuities and legacies in the way health care has been conducted and the success of educational innovations might well rely on their fitting into and adding value to this 'legacy'.

Equally, perhaps many innovations in communication skills so far have floundered because they have sought to introduce new practices and not taken into account the existing work that goes on in health care settings. While practitioners may well have absorbed the professional wisdom about the importance of communication in ensuring good outcomes for clients and themselves, they may well continue using timeworn communicative strategies of the kind that lead to complaints, poor outcomes and a sense of alienation between client and practitioner.

Hence, we would like to enter a plea which sounds remarkably simple but is often very difficult to put into practice. Look at what's already there. As one of the mid-20th century's great innovators in social science, Harvey Sacks, put it 'be interested in what you've got' (1992: 471). Rather than develop an overly detailed theoretical model of the health care encounter in advance, we prefer instead approaches which begin from ethnographic enquiry, painstaking recording and transcription, so as to achieve a thorough linguistic account of health care work (Garfinkel 1986; Crabtree et al. 2000). While it may appear strange to juxtapose the terms 'caring' and 'work', we do so in the sense that the 'liturgy of the clinic' (Atkinson 1995) is a linguistic or language dominant space full of ongoing practical activity: of admitting patients, conducting assessments, of taking temperatures, blood pressures and body fluid specimens, delivering diagnostic news, applying dressings and all the other mundane socially organized events that 'go on' in and 'make up' the health care environment, whether this be in the clinic or the client's home. This sense of ongoing practical activity means that the home or the clinic may be characterized as a site of 'work'. Once we begin examining this work it becomes clear that the work that takes place is part and parcel of, and elaborates, the health care legacy. Decisions as to whether grease or water is best applied to burns, or whether a minor wound merits a sticking plaster or whether an invalid should be kept warm or cool all depend on a kind of legacy, a commonsensical wisdom that can be traced back through the generations.

Sometimes the force of the legacy can be very powerful indeed. Ignaz Semmelweis was credited with the observation in 1846 that hand washing by the attending doctors could reduce the death rate of mothers and infants during childbirth dramatically. Medical students and doctors had previously gone straight from dissecting cadavers to attending births, perhaps wiping their hands on their aprons as they strode along the corridor. It was, thought Semmelweis, 'the examining finger which introduces the cadaveric particles' (Elek 1966: 349). His ideas were not popular at the time and he was dismissed from his post at the Vienna General Hospital. His subsequent writings were ignored and ridiculed, and he was reduced to distributing his ideas by means of pamphlets he handed out on the streets of Budapest – 'Beware of doctors, they will kill you'. Even this did not last long, as he was committed to an insane asylum in Vienna. 'He was not in the asylum for long. Thirteen days after admission he was dead'. He had been beaten to death. The autopsy report read: 'It is obvious that these horrible injuries were ... the consequences of brutal beating, tying down, trampling underfoot' (Carter et al. 1995: 260). It was difficult for his colleagues to accept that the physician could possibly be the cause of disease. The legacy in this case made innovation all but impossible. Now this is not necessarily the fate of all innovators in medicine. The example should show however that changing beliefs and practices can be hard work and sometimes involves considerable personal cost to the innovator.

But that is not all. Sometimes contemporary situational constraints on good practice may be just as recalcitrant. Hand washing in modern health care is sometimes little better than it was in Semmelweis's day, such that Albert and Condie (1981) discovered that intensive care-unit personnel washed their hands less than half the time, with physicians being 'the worst offenders'. 'Dry skin' and being 'too busy' were the most often used excuses in a study by Boyce (1999). In one Australian study, while doctors estimated their own hand washing rates at 50–95 per cent of encounters, observational evidence suggested that the rate was in fact 9 per cent (Tibballs 1996).

In the light of this, innovations and educational interventions to enhance health care need to be responsive to the constraints of everyday work. Innovators and educators should be sensitive to the self-serving tendencies in practitioners' and patients' own accounts. New technologies have to be embedded within these socially organized activities of the health care setting and their use will be constrained by these activities themselves. Social life in health care, despite the permanent revolution, crisis and chaos identified by many commentators, can be remarkably resistant to change.

The social order of health care: early theories and approaches

Social theorists who have turned their attention to health care settings have often been fascinated by this orderliness and ritualization which is often apparent. Hence, in the next section of the chapter we will consider some of the approaches that might be applied to the question, 'how is social order possible?' This is a classic sociological question and, in the context of this book, might better be put as 'how is social order possible in health care settings?'

One of the classic attempts to answer this came from Talcott Parsons (1951) who famously promoted the idea of a 'sick role'. As Turner (1992: 215) subsequently argued: 'Becoming sick requires the patient to learn how to perform according to certain norms of appropriate behaviour; there are appropriate and inappropriate rules of conduct which are expected of a person who has been correctly identified as "sick"'. Around the middle of the 20th century Talcott Parsons was interested in how people displayed sickness and how this affected their interaction with people around them. Parsons's classic formulation of the role involves four components:

(1) Sick individuals are exempted from their normal social responsibilities.
(2) Others accept that they cannot help being ill.
(3) They should want to get well.
(4) They should seek appropriate medical help to enable their recovery.

(1951: 436–7).

But there was more to it than simply a role. The experiences, actions and social processes were believed to affect their mental life too. As Turner points out, it combined 'elements of Freudian psychoanalysis with the sociological analysis of roles and a comparative cultural understanding of the importance of illness in industrial societies' (1992: 137). By combining Freud's theory of internal psychological organization with a functionalist theory of social structure, Parsons's understanding of the 'role' effectively combined micro and macro levels of analysis. This concept of the socialized 'sick role' allowed a model of the self to be constructed which was also informed by collective, structural norms and constraints. Even today, this remains an important insight into the social forces that shape medical encounters (Fahy and Smith 1999).

Parsons's notion of the sick role has been criticized on a number of counts. Just over ten years later Goffman published *Asylums* (1962) describing the coercive and dehumanizing regimes that could easily evolve in hospitals, challenging the implied agreement and accord which appeared to infuse Parsons's model. Moreover, the grounded focus of interactionist work such as Goffman's, which is full of observations and examples from his studies of hospital practice has formed the basis for a valuable critique of the empirical inadequacies of Parsons' work. Goffman's work was also ground breaking in that he argued that social order was negotiated and that exercises of authority by staff in hospitals could often be accompanied by acts of resistance by patients. Even so, Goffman's accounts of negotiated forms of self are somewhat difficult to relate to broader social patterns. Fahy and Smith (1999) see Goffman's work as being rooted in the American pragmatist tradition, a philosophical movement which is concerned with the relationship between meanings and actions. Interactionist accounts like Goffman's typically see patients' selves and identities as being created through 'illness action' and interaction. The identities which emerge do so as emergent properties of local, institutional situations and biographical experiences. This kind of perspective focuses on the local and particular and tends not to try to produce a powerful, synthetic generalizable model of how selves and identities are created that can be applied to differing institutional and cultural contexts.

Indeed, sometimes this is made a virtue by some researchers and theorists. In the case of conversation analysis, the local order of conversation is the primary social order, and possibly the only one worth thinking about. As Harvey Sacks put it, there is 'order at all points'. Moreover, as far as conversation analysts are concerned that's the only order there is. From this point of view

> the primordial site of social order is found in members' use of methodical practices to produce, make sense of and thereby render accountable, features of their local circumstances ... The socially structured character of ... any enterprise undertaken by members is thus not exterior or extrinsic to their everyday workings, but interior and intrinsic, residing in the local and particular detail of practical actions undertaken by members uniquely competent to do so.
>
> (Boden and Zimmerman 1991: 6–7)

Moreover, conversation analysis has its own epistemology (theory of knowledge) in that it does not concern itself with matters that are outside the conversation:

> No assumptions are made regarding the participants' motivations, intentions or purposes; nor about their ideas, thoughts or understandings; nor their moods, emotions or feelings, except insofar as these can demonstrably be shown to be matters that participants themselves are noticing, attending to or orienting to in the course of their interaction.
>
> (Psathas 1995: 47)

Conversation analytic approaches therefore tend to have the same squeamish attitude to thinking about the cognitive and emotional state of the participants and the larger-scale social structure (West 1984). While their strength lies in their focus on language and concrete micro-sequences of interaction as critical to maintaining medical power, these methods do not seek to understand the self, and the extracts of encounters they present have a curiously disembodied quality (Lynch and Bogen 1994).

This forms an important strand in research on health care, and one to which we shall return in Chapter 5. Following this approach, in a good many studies of health care encounters, the events are often described as the product of interactions and interactional competencies, with realities being constructed *in situ* by the interactants. Usually there is only minimal reference to the wider, extra-situational structural conditions shaping the identities of the people working through the encounters, and little systematic grasp of how health care encounters reproduce relations of power (Pappas 1990). Rather than broader propositions about the nature of medical power in encounters, interactionists are more usually concerned with methodological problems and procedures for assembling data (e.g. Denzin 1989).

By contrast, structural Marxist accounts of the medical encounter provide an almost exact opposite to interactionist models, stressing the way power might be exerted over health care encounters from superior to subordinate, from economy to social life and, lastly, to individual consciousness and action. Typically, these models involve the idea of a dominant ideology, in which the patient is trapped by discourses and procedures that compel obedience. As Fahy and Smith (1999) remind us, this kind of theorizing offers a robust model of power and social structure, but leaves us with little insight concerning agency, contingency or the self (Pappas 1990). In considering social structure and health it might consider how economic inequalities determine access to public health (Farmer 2003). In health care encounters, this kind of analysis might lead us to think about the economics and politics of how medicine is in thrall to the interests of large drug companies (e.g. Healy 2004). However, these analyses can be limiting as a way of thinking about health care encounters because they provide little room for theorizing either the shifting identities that run through interactions or the autonomy of culture.

Power: making sense of inequality in the health care encounter and the work of Michel Foucault

Growing dissatisfaction with functionalist and interactionist accounts in terms of how they address the issue of larger scale social power is perhaps one reason why Foucauldian approaches have provided an increasingly influential alternative for critical sociologists over the past ten years. Foucault and the post-structuralists draw our attention to the manner in which the reality we think we know is not essentially 'there' but is merely one of several possibilities that 'could be there'. What we see is the product of particular sets of power relationships. The implication is that under other sets of power relationships a very different reality could be produced. In the conventional view, clinics might exist to cure the patient and prisons might rehabilitate the criminal, but from a Foucauldian perspective we might equally say that the institutions and their associated discourses pin pathological identities – 'patient', 'invalid', 'criminal' – on socially marginalized people.

In Foucauldian analysis, the focus on institutional discourses and identities marks an important break with the class-based modes of analysis found in Marxism and structural functionalism. Instead it points towards a more local and cultural under-standing of how selves are constructed, positioned and aligned with the larger scale government of conduct and subjectivity (Foucault 1977; Rose 1990; Dean 1999). These authors have sought to understand how power works in subtle ways at the level of consciousness, personal identity and language, offering us a means of thinking about the repercussions of knowledge, policy and power at the individual level. Foucault (e.g. 1977, 1980, 1990) has been readily incorporated within scholarship on health care where authors have argued that these disciplines participate in regimes of truth such that the nature of realities – health, illness and treatment for example – are fundamentally social and textually mediated practices, rather than for example rely-ing solely on the scientific principles of medicine (Gastaldo and Holmes 1999).

Yet Foucault's approach is criticized for being relatively insensitive to questions of identity, struggle and contingency (Fraser 1989; Deveaux 1994). In Foucault's work one need only think of the concepts of the *panopticon* – Jeremy Bentham's famous circular prison – and the 'docile body' to see the overwhelming emphasis on mechanisms of conformity and control within the institution. What is left out of the frame here is not just struggle, 'resistance' and the subjective experience of dis-ciplinary power: 'Where there is power, there is resistance, and that however, or rather equally, the latter is never in a position of exteriority in relation to power' (Foucault 1990: 126–7). The occupying forces and the resistance are likely, in other words, to be singing from the same song sheet. There is also seldom any reference to wider socially structured human experiences and identities, systematic inequalities of gender, race and class, individual life-histories and so on, that have an impact upon particular encounters within health care (Deveaux 1994: 227).

In the 20 years since his death, Foucault has been enormously influential in the study of health care and his concepts will continually appear through the pages of this book. However, despite his wide appeal, there is a yearning for something that allows us to think more clearly about the possibility of autonomy, resistance, struggle and escape. As a blockbuster movie Foucault has no happy ending. Power, through its 'capillary' action, gets everywhere.

Critical linguistics and health care language

A somewhat different perspective is provided by the discipline of critical language study. Here, as with Foucault, there is a commitment to unmasking power differ-entials, yet it also contains a more liberatory ambition to make talk and text more emancipatory.

A good deal of language and communication study, whether of spoken or written discourse, is essentially a descriptive practice. It usually involves the analysis of texts in order to understand how and why they work in relation to the context in which they were produced. 'Critical language study' or 'critical discourse analysis' by contrast is explicitly concerned with analysing texts in terms of their relationship with societies and their institutions. In a sense critical approaches to the study of communication stem from the desire to analyse social phenomena, using texts as evidence of social trends, practices or norms worthy of further exploration. Critical discourse analysts, such as Norman Fairclough, see discourse as 'language as a form of social practice' and that 'language is part of society and not somehow external to it ... language is a social process ... and language is a socially conditioned process, conditioned that is by other non-linguistic parts of society' (1989: 22). Hence in critical discourse analysis the term 'discourse' takes on a much broader meaning and can refer to the whole process by which the language in question came to be produced. It reflects the sense-making activities of the speakers and writers but also the institutional norms and standards where it is created and used.

Fairclough's (1992) work draws a number of insights from the earlier literary theorist, Mikhail Bakhtin, in particular the idea that any utterance or text is inherently intertextual. That is, any one text can be seen to contain elements of others. Advertisements and music videos contain elements that remind us of feature films, conversations in doctor's surgeries resemble exchanges from medical dramas on television, advice about relationships in magazines recollects the insights from couples counselling – the list could go on. Any one text is made up of elements of another. According to Fairclough discourse may involve 'manifest intertextuality' – direct quotations for example – or 'constitutive intertextuality (or interdiscursivity)', where one genre or discourse type uses the textual features of another apparently unrelated genre.

As a result of this grafting, borrowing and poaching aspect of language, it is not surprising that discursive practices are changing, and critical discourse analysis accords a central place to the recognition of how textual features from one genre, say private, informal conversation, might appear in other genres, for example medical consultations.

Once we note this intertextuality, this then poses further questions about why the language is being used in this way and whose interests it serves. For example, why might a doctor try to adopt the style of an adult talking to a child when examining a patient? Why might managers in the health service adopt the style of a casual acquaintance when talking to their clinical colleagues? Fairclough (1992, 2003) argued that an important element of social change in many developed societies involves changes in the ways in which people use language. However, relationships between managers and staff are not necessarily any more equitable. It is merely that the asymmetry is disguised. Informality may be a disguise to coerce staff into carrying out more tasks. Indeed, with an increasingly casualized labour force the power of managers over their junior colleagues' livelihoods has perhaps increased. When a doctor speaks to a patient informally, to what extent does this indicate that the patient has been 'empowered'? Or is this a mere token concession to the idea that the patient is in control of their own treatment? As David Smail (2005) remarks, the 'empowered' are not necessarily the same as the powerful. These are the type of questions that a critical analyst would ask.

Despite this apparent democratization, health care language is still frequently dominated by medical concerns. For example, Wadensten (2005) reports upon the morning conversations between staff and elderly residents in a nursing home. Despite their conversational style, it is noteworthy that 89 per cent of the recorded events were primarily about health and sickness, reflecting the biomedical 'frame' of the nurses. This suggests that some power of the institution or the professionals within it was still at work to determine the content of the conversations, especially as the vast majority of them were initiated by nurses themselves.

The theme of power is one to which we shall return later in this book, as the study of health communication has had a persistent concern with power. In contemporary policy discourse there is a great deal of discussion of client or patient 'empowerment'. This appears in the UK's *NHS Plan* (Department of Health 2000) and more recently the idea of 'empowering and mobilizing communities' has appeared in *Shaping the Future of Public Health* (Department of Health 2005b). Yet as Graham (2004) cautions, empowerment as a guiding philosophy in health and social care is largely defined by professionals. The theoretical traditions of Marxist, Foucauldian and critical discourse scholarship outlined earlier can assist in probing within the understandings of this contested conceptual ideal and, as Graham (2004) notes, we might reveal that the socio-cultural perspectives of the oppressed communities that it claims to address have instead been sidelined or excluded.

Extending the focus on language, identity and power: Judith Butler and the performances of health care

To help us understand health care encounters further, and link them to the broader society of which they are a part let us now turn to a strand of scholarship that has less frequently been applied to health care but nevertheless might be useful in revealing some insights about the way that people conduct themselves in health care settings. This next perspective draws on postmodernism and some aspects of language theory and we believe it has a great deal of potential in this field. This is what we might call 'performative theory' and was originally set in motion by Judith Butler (1990a) who considered gender to be a kind of 'performative'. But the origins of the idea go even further back – Butler borrowed the idea from linguistics, especially Austin's (1962) early forays into speech act theory. Thus to say that a statement, a story about oneself or a display of healthy or sick behaviour is a 'performative' is to say that it is bringing something into being. In this view, describing the hardship of suffering a disease, the satisfaction of caring work, or the conflict between home and working life as a service provider is not simply to describe a fact of male or female experience, it is to do with how the speaker is knowingly assembling an identity as a person with certain moral qualities.

Butler (1990b) thus offers what she herself calls 'a more radical use of the doctrine of constitution that takes the social agent as an *object* rather than the subject of constitutive acts' (p. 270). Butler argues that we cannot even assume a stable subjectivity that goes about performing various roles; rather, it is the very act of performing that constitutes who we are. Butler originally formulated these ideas in relation to gender but they might equally well be applicable to performing the role and duties of a patient or health professional. Identity itself, for Butler, is an illusion created by our performances. The belief in stable gender identities, health care identities and gendered experiences of health and illness is, Butler might argue, compelled 'by social sanction and taboo'.

Butler's idea that power processes control how we acquire identity might perhaps also help us understand how people assume identities as patients, nurses or doctors (Fahy and Smith 1999). The process of identification enables some identities and closes off others. The formation of identity involves the fear of punishment if one does not comply with the rules of the game as a 'good patient' or 'caring nurse' for example, and encompasses language and symbols, including the body itself, and is reproduced in interaction.

What is more interesting is what happens to those who are not on the right path and who do not inhabit the highly valued ends of the binaries. Many of us, according to Butler (1993), have our range of possible identities foreclosed through fear of 'abjection'. Butler's use of the concept of 'abjection' denotes something akin to pollution: that which is dirty or corrupt and must be kept out of sight; a degraded or cast out status. This abject domain is a site of dreaded identifications bringing with it the fear of a symbolic death so that the subject would give up their autonomy rather than face abjection (p. 3). The abject domain has many parallels with the roles and identities of participants in the field of health care – the person with AIDS (Larson 2005), the person experiencing homelessness, the intravenous drug user. Rather than seeing the subject as 'choosing' to assume a subject position Butler (1993:2) argues that power generates this identification, abjection and subjectivity. Once an individual takes up an identification or subject position there is a particular discourse which belongs to that identity. Someone whose health problems are linked to their recreational drug use will mobilize a different set of discourses than someone injured during a rugby match.

This way of thinking about health care encounters enables us to make sense of the role of social structure and social inequality. The distribution of powerful subject positions, and their composition, corresponds with the distribution of social power more widely and tends to operate so as to reproduce this power. In the case of gender, the range of positions available to women – often based upon traditional, socially prescribed subject positions – centred upon a moral ethic of care (Ring 1994). Fahy and Smith (1999: 85) describe, for example a young woman having a difficult and painful labour and wishing to have an assisted delivery with increased anesthesia. She was told by a doctor, 'There is no reason that you should not have a normal delivery. You are just being selfish. Because of your selfishness the baby could be injured, even brain damaged. I'll have to ask the consultant about that'. Such an ethic of selflessness demands the suppression of one's own needs, sometimes to the point of self-martyrdom.

This idea of identity being closely bound up with performance and action is common not only to Butler's theory of selves and identities, but to other traditions in social theory too. The sense of an identity or a role as a scripted performance is one way of looking at it, but equally there is a good deal of creative improvization too. It is in this context that the work of French sociologist and philosopher, Pierre Bourdieu, is perhaps particularly relevant to the study of health care communication. His work has been strangely absent from much health care scholarship so far. This is unfortunate, for, as we hope to show, Bourdieu's research offers a fine 'critical' yet reflexive vantage point from which to view the organized social practices of health care.

Field, habitus and doxa: the relevance of Pierre Bourdieu to health care studies

In much of his work, Bourdieu invites us to attend to symbolic structures, and to consider their relation to both the cognitive and emotional structures of the individual and social structures of society. Particularly relevant to our purposes, he draws our attention to language, categorizations and labels, and their systems of production and mode of consumption. These he feels are critical in the reproduction and transformation of the social world. Three major assumptions run through Bourdieu's work (Bourdieu and Wacquant 1992: 12–14). First, he believes that individuals' mental schemata are a kind of embodiment of social divisions, distinctions and categorizations. In other words, the social and the cognitive are inextricably linked. Thus, an analysis of social phenomena and structures logically carries through into an analysis of objective dispositions. Second, this correspondence between social and mental structures serves important political functions. It means that symbolic systems can be instruments of domination, not simply instruments of knowledge. This is aligned with many critiques of the power of medical care which see the very act of diagnosis – 'a destructive gift of difference' – as driving a wedge between professionals and those they seek to serve (Hayne 2003: 722). The categories with which the social world is perceived, imposing themselves 'with all appearances of objective necessity' (Bourdieu and Wacquant 1992: 13), decisively reinforce the social order. Accepting the idea that symbolic systems are social products that constitute social relations, Bourdieu suggests that to some extent one can transform the world by transforming its representation, to some extent. Following from this is Bourdieu's third main assumption: systems of classification are sites of struggle between individuals and groups. Social taxonomies such as ethnic groups, occupations, illnesses, treatments and so on are the result of and at stake in social power relations. It becomes important therefore to consider how language and, more broadly, 'symbolic goods' contribute to the reproduction and transformation of structures of domination. Consider this account of a psychiatrist, 'Errol', at work:

> The patients were treated with a courteous benevolence, like good dogs. It was astonishing to see how, being treated with total authoritarian objectivity, they responded with total submissive gratitude. Errol gave the impression of being absolutely *sure*. While he was sure about everything, he addressed but one thing: drugs. If his patients wanted to talk diagnosis, he talked drugs. If they wanted to talk symptoms, he talked drugs. Stress? Drugs. Suffering? Drugs. Family problems? Drugs. Job? Drugs. The love his patients felt for Errol was palpable. How could they love him? They could love him because not only did he convey to them that he was sure about their drugs, and by implication about all the other things they mentioned, but in addition he always said to each patient at the end of the ten-minute interview: 'This will make you feel wonderful and make you *better*.' Most patients loved hearing this and thanked him. A rare patient might ask 'Are you sure?' 'Absolutely. This will make you feel wonderful and make you *better*.'
>
> (Shem 1999: 743)

This, in slightly sensationalized terms, is a part of caring work. The clients' difficulties are transformed into something that the health care professional can tackle according to the concepts, theories and treatments available. But what is also apparent to Shem as a naïve observer is that power is at work here – not only the institutional and personal power of the psychiatrist but also the power of symbolic capital in the form of knowledge of psychopharmacology. Whether or not it was literally true that the patients would improve on the drugs was less important. What was more important is the concordance achieved between doctor and patient that this is a good course of action, as a result of the doctor's symbolic power.

Bourdieu's (1999) theory of power draws heavily on notions of 'symbolic power' and 'symbolic capital'. This refers to the social value attributed to certain things, whether they are knowledge, practice, economic resources or political power. According to Bourdieu, there are different forms of capital in society, including economic (or material) capital, cultural capital, symbolic capital and linguistic capital and this forms a useful backdrop against which to think about governmentality in clinical settings.

The medical discourse then constitutes a form of symbolic capital, of a kind that has been imbued with status and value as Thornborrow (2002: 6) notes; those who deploy the most powerful form of cultural capital are advantaged: 'Knowledge of and access to those practices put some people in potentially more powerful positions than others'. Individual practitioners may learn the appropriate choreography to perform with the key terms in order to accrue capital for themselves so that they can become 'competent' and 'successful' clinicians within the health care facility. In this view, it is through language that power relationships are acted out: 'linguistic exchanges are also relations of symbolic power in which the power relations between speakers or their respective groups are actualized' (Bourdieu 1991: 37).

There are three further concepts of Bourdieu's which deserve elaboration in this context and which may well allow us to make sense of health care. The first is that of the 'field', a set of social relations within which the social drama is played out, the second is the 'habitus', which describes the mode of conduct of the social actors, and the third is 'doxa' or the rules of the game in which the actors are involved.

Field

Fields, according to Bourdieu (1990), are 'networks of social relations, structured systems of social positions within which struggles or manoeuvres take place over resources, stakes and access'. Scheuer (2003: 145) adds a definition of a 'field' as 'a structured network of social practices and positions related to a trade or area of production'. Therefore, different health care practitioners can be perceived as occupying different fields depending upon how much capital they have acquired through the amount of prestigious language and social practice that they are able to perform. Chouliaraki and Fairclough (1999) argue that Bourdieu's decision to differentiate between fields enables 'empirical investigation of shifts in the social practices of late modernity' to be conducted (p. 101), which is aligned with our aim of examining the shifting communicative patterns of health care. Fields are occupied by two sets of actors, the dominant and the dominated who attempt to usurp, exclude, and establish monopoly over the mechanisms of the field's reproduction and the type of power effective in it (p. 106). Fields are dynamic social microcosms, forever-changing, and require a study approach that recognizes their relational or dialectical qualities (p. 96). The field, then, comprises the social totality of the relevant actors (DiMaggio and Powell 1983: 149), not simply what occurs 'within the health care encounter' or 'within the profession'. Furthermore, when one comes to think in terms of field, the focus turns to power, domination and class. One might suggest, as does Drummond (1998), that health care organizations are best seen as subfields, or as embedded in a larger field, and are enclosed in a social universe with its own laws of functioning. This enables us to see the health care setting, like a field, as a space in which a game takes place, or as a field of relations between individuals who are competing for personal or own-group advantage.

Habitus

The players in the field are not simply infinitely re-transforming themselves according to where their advantage lies. They play according to a personal disposition or 'habitus'. This is their characteristic style of play which enables them to be recognized by what they say, do, wear or how they carry themselves. Habitus is the 'durably inculcated system of structured, structuring dispositions' found within a field (Bourdieu 1990: 52). Habitus is embodied within individual social actors. It is 'the social inscribed in the body ... a feel for or sense of the "social game" ... the source of most practices ... a tendency to generate regulated behaviours apart from any reference to rules' (Bourdieu 1962: 111). Habitus exists in the form of mental and corporeal schemata, a matrix of perception, appreciation and action (Bourdieu and Wacquant 1992: 16–18). In short, habitus saturates social processes (Foster 1986: 105). One might have the habitus of a nurse or a doctor, or a patient, care assistant, carer or relative. Sometimes this is explicitly advised but most often, however, it is assumed naturally, as if this were the only way to speak, think and behave.

Like a field, habitus is not static, being a combination of the social actor's more deeply ingrained identity with his or her more transient identities as a health professional, patient, student, parent and so on (Meisenhelder 1997). The habitus is also always changing because it is constantly exposed to new experiences, many of which are reinforcing, but often modify it over a period of time (Bourdieu and Wacquant 1992: 133). Habitus also changes because of changes in the climate of the field, and in the kinds of capital available and the struggles over them. Even apparently trivial aspects of health care life make sense in this framework. The notorious illegibility of doctors' handwriting may be more than just accidental. Medical students may actually 'gain advantage from illegibility' (Kandela 1999). Illegible handwriting may also represent a symbol of superiority: 'My time is more valuable than yours', it says. 'You can take the time to decipher what I write' (Winslow 1997).

Although society may be 'in the individual as the habitus' (Meisenhelder 1997: 180), habitus is also constitutive of the field, working in a dialectic fashion, as an infinite yet strictly limited generative capacity, as determinism and freedom, as conditioning and creativity, and as consciousness and the unconscious (Bourdieu 1990: 55). As Bourdieu (1988: 784) notes: 'The field, as a structured space, tends to structure the habitus, while the habitus tends to structure the perceptions of the field'. Habitus may appear in differing ways: as a 'collective habitus' – a unifying cultural code; a 'dispositional habitus' – an internalized cultural code; or as a 'manifest habitus' the practice of a characteristic style (Nash 1990: 434).

Despite the fact that the people involved are not necessarily aware of what they are doing, in this view social agents are not merely objects guided by rules or codes. However, Bourdieu argues that social agents pursue strategies and weigh their 'interests' prior to any action. It is merely that these strategies are always in some way constrained by field and habitus. For example, as reported by Macklin (1993) US newspapers reported that all obstetricians in a large region of Georgia came to an agreement that they would no longer provide obstetrical services to women who were lawyers, married to lawyers, or worked in any capacity in a law firm. Here we can see the relationship between changes in 'habitus' and changes in the 'field', as American culture became increasingly litigious and the symbolic power or legal knowledge of some patients – and the likelihood that they would use this against doctors – made them a risk not worth taking.

Doxa: the rules of the game

Another of Bourdieu's key terms that seems particularly pertinent to the exploration of the formation of sensibilities about health care is his notion of 'doxa', or the participant's 'commitment to the presuppositions' of the game that they are playing (1990: 66), an 'undisputed, pre-reflexive, naïve, native compliance' (p. 68) that gives us our 'feel' for what is, among other things, intuitively proper, fair, excellent or prestigious. Bourdieu adds that competitors in political power struggles often seek to appropriate 'the sayings of the tribe' (doxa) and thereby to appropriate 'the power the group exercises over itself' (p. 110; Wacquant 1999).

Conclusion: theories, evidence and social change

In this chapter then we have attempted to give the reader some sense of how communicative encounters in health care can be placed within a theoretical context. This might seem a little removed from the serious business of health care communication itself as it happens in the community or the clinic, but it is important to have a sense of how these encounters fit into a broader social whole. After all, very often when we study health care communication it is because, somewhere along the line, we want to change it. We may want to stop care staff talking to nursing home residents as if they were babies. We may want patients to be able to make informed choices. Perhaps we want to empower socially marginalized groups, or as policymakers we want to use the health care system to forward some goal such as 'social inclusion' or facilitate large-scale improvements in public health. It is therefore important to have a sense of how health care works and how it makes sense in society. Governments may create multiple policies for public and professional consumption, but unless policymakers have a clear vision of how societies work it is doubtful whether any consistent improvement can be achieved.

Many of the perspectives we have covered here do not necessarily make predictions that can be tested in experimental settings. Rather, they provide a way of looking at the world, a sensitizing perspective or an array of concepts with which the social world of health care can be interrogated. They are concepts to which we shall return in subsequent chapters as we attempt to place the question of evidence-based communication in health care on some sort of theoretical footing.

References

Albert, R.K. and Condie, F. (1981) Hand-washing patterns in medical intensive-care units, *New England Journal of Medicine*, 304: 1465–6.

Atkinson, P. (1995) *Medical Talk and Medical Work: The Liturgy of the Clinic*. London: Sage.

Austin, J.L. (1962) *How to Do Things with Words*. Oxford: Clarendon Press.

Boden, D. and Zimmerman, D.H. (1991) *Talk and Social Structure: Studies in Ethnomethodology and Conversation Analysis*. Cambridge: Polity Press.

Bolton, G. (2005) Medicine and literature: writing and reading, *Journal of Evaluation in Clinical Practice*, 11(2): 171–9.

Boyce, J.M. (1999) It is time for action: improving hand hygiene in hospitals, *Annals of Internal Medicine*, 130: 153–5.

Bourdieu, P. (1962) *The Algerians*. Boston: Beacon.

Bourdieu, P. (1988) Vive la crise! For heterodoxy in social science, *Theory and Society*, 17: 773–87.

Bourdieu, P. (1990) *The Logic of Practice*. Cambridge: Polity Press.

Bourdieu, P. (1991) *Language and Symbolic Power*. Cambridge: Polity Press.

Bourdieu, P. (1999) *Outline of a Theory of Practice*. Cambridge: Polity Press.

Bourdieu, P. and Wacquant, L.J.D. (eds) (1992) *An Invitation to Reflexive Sociology*. Chicago: University of Chicago Press.

Brown, B., Crawford, P. and Hicks, C. (2003) *Evidence-based Research*. Buckingham: Open University Press.

Burnard, P. (2003) Ordinary chat and therapeutic conversation: phatic communication and mental health nursing, *Journal of Psychiatric and Mental Health Nursing*, 10: 678–82.

Butler, J. (1990a) *Gender Trouble: Feminism and the Subversion of Identity*. London: Routledge.

Butler, J. (1990b) Performative acts and gender constitution: an essay in phenomenology and feminist theory, in S.E. Case (ed.) *Performing Feminisms: Feminist Critical Theory and Theatre*. Baltimore, MD: Johns Hopkins University Press.

Butler, J. (1993) *Bodies That Matter*. New York: Routledge.

Carter, K.S., Abbott, S. and Siebach, J.L. (1995) Five documents relating to the final illness and death of Ignaz Semmelweis, *Bulletin of the History of Medicine*, 69: 255–70.

Chouliaraki, L. and Fairclough, N. (1999) *Discourse in Late Modernity: Re-thinking Critical Discourse Analysis*. Edinburgh: Edinburgh University Press.

Crabtree, A. (2003) *Designing Collaborative Systems: A Practical Guide to Ethnography*. London: Springer-Verlag.

Crabtree, A., O'Brien, J., Nichols, D., Rouncefield, M. and Twidale, M. (2000) Ethnomethodologically informed ethnography and information systems design, *Journal of the American Society for Information Science*, 51(7): 666–82.

Das Gupta, S. (2003) Reading bodies, writing bodies: self-reflection and cultural criticism in a narrative medicine curriculum, *Literature and Medicine*, 22(2): 241–56.

Davies, N. (2000) Patients' and carers' perceptions of factors influencing recovery after cardiac surgery, *Journal of Advanced Nursing*, 32(2): 318–26.

Dean, M. (1999) *Governmentality: Power and Rule in Modern Society*. London: Sage.

Denzin, N. (1989) *Interpretive Interactionism*. Newbury Park, CA: Sage.

Department of Health (2000) *The NHS Plan: A Plan for Investment, a Plan for Reform*. London: Stationery Office.

Department of Health (2005a) *Tackling Health Inequalities: Status Report on the Programme for Action*. London: Department of Health.

Department of Health (2005b) *Shaping the Future of Public Health: Promoting Health in the NHS*. London: Department of Health.

Deveaux, M. (1994) Feminism and empowerment, *Feminist Studies*, 20(2): 223–47.

DiMaggio, P. and Powell, W.W. (1983) The iron cage revisited: institutional isomorphism and collective rationality in organizational fields, *American Sociological Review*, 48: 147–60.

Drummond, G. (1998) New theorizing about organizations: the emergence of narrative and social theory for management, *Current Topics in Management*, 3: 93–122.

Edmondson, R. (2003) Social capital: a strategy for enhancing health? *Social Science and Medicine*, 57: 1723–33.

Elek, S.D. (1966) Semmelweis and the Oath of Hippocrates, *Proceedings of the Royal Society of Medicine*, 59: 346–52.

Fahy, K. and Smith, P. (1999) From the sick role to subject positions: a new approach to the medical encounter, *Health*, 3(1): 71–93.

Fairclough, N. (1989) *Language and Power*. New York: Longman.

Fairclough, N. (1992) *Discourse and Social Change*. Cambridge: Polity Press.

Fairclough, N. (2003) *Analysing Discourse: Textual Analysis for Social Research*. London: Routledge.

Farmer, P. (2003) *Pathologies of Power: Health, Human Rights, and the New War on the Poor*. Berkeley, CA: University of California Press.

Foster, S. (1986) Reading Pierre Bourdieu, *Cultural Anthropology*, 1(1): 103–10.

Foucault, M. (1977) *Discipline and Punish: The Birth of the Prison*. Harmondsworth: Penguin.

Foucault, M. (1980) *Michel Foucault: Power/Knowledge – Selected Interviews and Other Writings 1972/1977*. Brighton: Harvester Wheatsheaf.

Foucault, M. (1990) *The History of Sexuality, Vol. 1: An Introduction*. Harmondsworth: Penguin.

Fraser, N. (1989) *Unruly Practices*. Minneapolis, MN: University of Minnesota Press.

Frid, I., Ohlen, J. and Bergbom, I. (2000) On the use of narratives in nursing research, *Journal of Advanced Nursing*, 32(3): 695–703.

Garfinkel, H. (ed.) (1986) *Ethnomethodological Studies of Work*. London: Routledge and Kegan Paul.

Gastaldo, D. and Holmes, D. (1999) Foucault and nursing: a history of the present, *Nursing Inquiry*, 6(4): 231–40.

Goffman, E. (1962) *Asylums*. Chicago: Aldine.

Goldstein, K., Kielhofner, G. and Paul-Ward, A. (2004) Occupational narratives and the therapeutic process, *Australian Occupational Therapy Journal*, 51:119–24.

Graham, M. (2004) Empowerment revisited: social work, resistance and agency in black communities, *European Journal of Social Work*, 7(1): 43–56.

Hayne, Y.M. (2003) Experiencing psychiatric diagnosis: client perspectives on being named mentally ill, *Journal of Psychiatric and Mental Health Nursing*, 10: 722–9.

Healy, D. (2004) *The Creation of Psychopharmacology*. Cambridge, MA.: Harvard University Press.

Kandela, P. (1999) Doctor's handwriting, *Lancet*, 353: 1109.

Kasper, G. (1997) *Can Pragmatic Competence be Taught?* (NetWork no. 6). Honolulu, HI: Second Language Teaching Curriculum Center, University of Hawaii.

Larson, S. (2005) New avenues for the politics of the abject, *American Literary History*, 17(3): 550–2.

Lynch, M. and Bogen, D. (1994) Harvey Sacks's primitive natural science, *Theory, Culture and Society*, 11: 65–104.

Macklin, R. (1993) *Enemies of Patients*. New York: Oxford University Press.

Meisenhelder, T. (1997) Pierre Bourdieu and the call for a reflexive sociology, *Current Perspectives in Social Theory*, 17: 159–83.

Mitchell, W.J. (2000) *e-topia*. Cambridge, MA.: MIT Press.

Nash, R. (1990) Bourdieu on education and social and cultural reproduction, *British Journal of Sociology of Education*, 11(4): 431–47.

Nelson, S. and McGillion, M. (2004) Expertise or performance? Questioning the rhetoric of contemporary narrative use in nursing, *Journal of Advanced Nursing*, 47(6): 631–8.

Pappas, G. (1990) Some implications for the study of doctor–patient interaction, *Social Science and Medicine*, 30(2): 199–204.

Parsons, T. (1951) *The Social System*. London: Routledge and Kegan Paul.

Peplau, H.E. (1952) *Interpersonal Relations in Nursing*. New York: G.P. Putnam's Sons.

Peplau, H.E. (1964) *Basic Principles of Patient Counselling*. Philadelphia, PA: Smith Kline and French Laboratories.

Psathas, G. (1995) *Conversation Analysis: The Study of Talk in Interaction*. London: Sage.

Ring, L. (1994) Sexual harassment and the production of gender, *Differences: A Journal of Feminist Cultural Studies*, 6(1): 129–66.

Rose, N. (1990) *Governing the Soul: The Shaping of the Private Self*. London: Routledge.

Rowe, R.E., Garcia, J., Macfarlane, A.J. and Davidson, L.L. (2001) Does poor communication contribute to stillbirths and infant deaths? A review, *Journal of Public Health Medicine*, 23: 23–34.

Sacks, H. (1992) (G. Jefferson, ed.) *Lectures on Conversation*. Oxford: Blackwell.

Scheuer, J. (2003) Habitus as the principle for social practice, *Language in Society*, 32(2): 143–75.

Schouten, B.C., Hoogstraten, J. and Eijkman, M.A.J. (2003) Patient participation during dental consultations: the influence of patients' characteristics and dentists' behaviour, *Community Dentistry and Oral Epidemiology*, 31(5): 368–77.

Shaw, M., Davey-Smith, G. and Dorling, D. (2005) Health inequalities and New Labour: how the promises compare with real progress, *British Medical Journal*, 330: 1016–21.

Shem, S. (1999) Mount misery, *British Medical Journal*, 318: 743.

Smail, D. (2005) *Power, Interest and Psychology: Elements of a Social, Materialist Understanding of Distress*. Ross on Wye: PCCS Books.

Taylor, C. (2003) Narrating practice: reflective accounts and the textual construction of reality, *Journal of Advanced Nursing*, 42(3): 244–51.

Thornborrow, J. (2002) *Power Talk: Language and Interaction in Institutional Discourse*. London: Longman.

Tibballs, J. (1996) Teaching medical staff to handwash, *Medical Journal of Australia*, 164: 395.

Turner, B. (1992) *Regulating Bodies*. London: Routledge.

Wadensten, B. (2005) The content of morning time conversations between nursing home staff and residents, *Journal of Clinical Nursing*, 14(8b): 84–9.

West, C. (1984) *Routine Complications*. Bloomington, IN: Indiana University Press.

Winslow, E.H. (1997) Legibility and completeness of physicians' handwritten medication orders, *Heart and Lung*, 26: 158–63.

2 The language of evidence: communicating about evidence in health care

Evidence-based practice: making sense of the debate

The concepts of evidence and evidence-based practice have been cornerstones of health care education for over a decade but they are still not proceeding as rapidly as some enthusiasts would wish. This impatience with the process of change can even be seen in fields like drug research, where randomized controlled clinical trials predominate. Thus, the status of evidence-based practice in the field of communication is perhaps even more fraught. In this chapter we cannot easily provide a neat set of evidence-based guidelines, but we hope that the reader will at least have some idea what the fuss is all about and why the issue provokes some strong feelings.

In order to make sense of the debates around evidence-based practice and health care communication, we will begin therefore with an examination of what constitutes evidence-based practice, and discuss the genealogy of the idea and its relevance to health care communication. For example, we will examine how it is that the whole idea of evidence-based health care has come to be seen by so many as anathema to client-centred and interpersonal approaches to care. The impatience on the part of enthusiasts for evidence-based practice with arguments that there are aspects of care which are somehow ineffable, numinous or beyond the grasp of scientific enquiry is almost palpable. Yet the equally persuasive argument that there are therapeutically significant aspects of communication and caring that are difficult to ensnare with experimental methods shows no sign of abating as the 21st century unfolds.

Rather than merely reproduce this polarized debate, we will try in this volume to instead identify points of contact and commonality between the two cultures of health care enquiry, thus pointing the way towards reconciliation of the viewpoints and research approaches. This issue also concerns the process of communication among health care educators, trainee practitioners and professionals themselves as they discuss evidence, establish the nature of the problems and identify how evidence might help them solve problems. The evidence-based practice ethos in health care has involved an increasing number of people in the health care workforce becoming research literate, yet the extent to which this means that health care is becoming evidence-based remains debatable.

In this chapter we will not merely be describing evidence about 'what works' in health care communication. What we will be doing instead is trying to think about how we conceptualize evidence and how we might bring this to bear on the health care encounter. It is in this way that we hope to get a little closer to the ideal of 'evidence-based communication' of this volume's title.

The 1990s and early 21st century have seen much debate about 'evidence-based policy and practice'. The veteran researcher and writer on gender issues, Ann Oakley, notes that this resembles a similar enterprise which burgeoned in the USA from the 1960s to the 1980s, and that the current move to evidence-based policy is paralleled by 'evidence-based medicine, evidence-based education, evidence-based social work, evidence-based policy making and evidence-based practice ... evidence-based everything' (2000: 308). Increasingly in the UK official statements about a broad range of helping professions assume evidence-based criteria as a building block of practice (see, *inter alia*, Audit Commission 1996; ESRC 2001).

As we will propose in this volume, a mutual interrogation between the study of interpersonal, communicative practice on the one hand and the tenets of evidence-based medicine on the other has important implications for the enrichment of both fields of enquiry.

There are several ways in which we could proceed. The first and most obvious is to go down a didactic path, which would involve laying out the kinds of evidence-based 'good practice' which are deemed to be desirable. There are at present a number of sources of this advice, with neat bullet-pointed lists about the importance of maintaining appropriate eye contact, asking open-ended questions, not interrupting the client at important points in their narrative, being polite and allowing the client to feel that he or she has been listened to. This kind of pedagogically oriented account of evidence-based practice has been attempted already. We shall follow a second and more challenging route. That is, in this chapter we shall try to encourage a different kind of understanding of 'evidence', 'practice' and their possible relationship.

At the time of writing, it must be admitted that the scope for new understanding and reconciliation between different camps in the debate does not look very likely. The evidence-based medicine rhetoric can sometimes sound less like the voice of dispassionate science than some kind of political posturing, aligning itself with the prevailing agendas of health care politics and economics in late modernity. Likewise, there is an implacable determination on the part of some scholars to insist that the process of care – interpersonal, holistic or spiritual – is beyond the reach of evidence-based metrics and measurements. In any case, the hope of a level playing field for such a debate is increasingly distant as it is tilted by a variety of secular and spiritual forces, which are variously governmental, commercial and populist. Concerns that drug companies are setting the scientific agenda of scholarly life in health care (Kmietowicz 2005) jostle with an increasing interest in complementary and alternative medicine (Marwick 2005) and a lingering suspicion that socioeconomic factors, rather than communicative ones, determine mortality and morbidity (Smith et al. 1997).

In such a climate also, it is difficult to theorize about the role of social, cultural and political systems, for they may be denigrated as unscientific (Larner 2004). Under a purportedly rational economic regime, governments, health care providers, research councils and academic institutions jockey for their share of the evidence-based pie, where using quantitative methods, statistical analyses and best of all, randomized controlled trials, is believed to guarantee the originator a more advantageous place at the funding table.

Evidence-based practice and the study of health care communication

At the time of writing, the situation in most developed nations still closely resembles Bensing's characterization at the turn of the century:

> Modern medicine is dominated by two general beliefs or paradigms: one is called 'evidence-based medicine'; the other is called 'patient-centered medicine'. Both concepts are generally accepted as 'good', 'valuable', and something to strive for. Few people will deny the relevance of either of them. But two serious questions can be raised. How patient-centered is evidence-based medicine? And, how evidence-based is patient-centered medicine? Close inspection of the literature reveals that evidence-based medicine and patient-centered medicine seem to belong to separate worlds.
>
> (2000: 17–18)

Thus, there are a number of key players in the UK who demur from the blanket imposition of an evidence-based framework that relies heavily on experiments. Greenhalgh (1999: 323) argues that: 'Clinical method is an interpretive act which draws on narrative skills to integrate the overlapping stories told by patients, clinicians and test results'. As Larner (2004: 31) adds, 'Therapists, like doctors, need to know what works in practice, how to best help a person, and research shows working with personal narrative and relational context is integral to the healing process'.

In the light of this, the exhortations to employ evidence-based practice can seem very hard-nosed indeed. Through the 1990s there occurred a 'paradigm shift' in health care in which the promotion of evidence-based medicine 'de-emphasize[d] intuition, unsystematic clinical experience, and pathophysiologic rationale' in clinical decision making, and stressed instead 'the examination of evidence from clinical research' (Evidence-based Medicine Working Group 1992: 2420–1). This privileging of comparative, experimental research evidence as the most credible source of knowledge for clinical practice was met with some scepticism by many practitioners. Since the inception of this new era of evidence-based health care there has been much debate about the factors that contribute to clinical excellence, what the limitations are of clinical research based on a model of randomized controlled trials and what the appropriate factors are that need to be considered in clinical decision making (see Miles et al. 2002).

The definition of evidence-based practice by Sackett et al. (1996: 71) still commands considerable assent among practitioners and researchers. It is 'the conscientious, explicit and judicious use of current best evidence in making decisions about the care of individual patients, based on the skills which allow the doctor [sic] to evaluate both personal experience and external evidence in a systematic and objective manner'.

Here, for example, is the kind of typology of evidence presented by the UK's Department of Health (1996). In descending order of credibility it includes:

1. Strong evidence from at least one systematic review of multiple well-designed randomized controlled trials.
2. Strong evidence from at least one properly designed randomized controlled trial of appropriate size.
3. Evidence from well-designed trials such as non-randomized trials, cohort studies, time series or matched case-controlled studies.
4. Evidence from well-designed non-experimental studies from more than one centre or research group.
5. Opinions of respected authorities, based on clinical evidence, descriptive studies or reports of expert committees.

Thus, the only thing better than a randomized controlled trial is a large number of these which are sufficiently similar that their data (or perhaps some measure of effect size) can be added together in a meta-analysis or systematic review. This then is the evidence on which practitioners are encouraged to base their work.

As we have noted elsewhere (Brown et al. 2003), the arguments in favour of evidence-based practice are commonsensically persuasive on scientific, humanitarian and politico-economic grounds. As we have also said before, however (Crawford et al. 2002), there appears to be a widespread assumption that we can change the culture of the health care professions by educating practitioners in the ways of evidence-based health care. This has led to much pedagogic innovation, but progress is still slower than some enthusiasts would wish, especially when it comes to embedding evidence-based health care in practice. As we discovered, while it is said to be desirable, people often find a whole range of good reasons why they cannot employ evidence-based practice, as a result of time and access constraints or because the issues with which they are dealing have not, they say, been specifically dealt with in the research literature (Crawford et al. 2002). In some cases also practitioners are unsure where to look or state that their work in community contexts means they cannot spend all day in the library or on a computer. In addition to the acknowledged presence of these practical and cultural constraints, as Larner (2004: 32) adds, 'The science of therapy is a creative, artful process where evidence about what works best for whom is applied to the person's story'.

Closing the gap between communicative action and evidence-based health care

As we suggested earlier, evidence for what works best in terms of communication is problematic. But we can begin our enquiry by examining the roles of communication in health care. According to Widder (2004: 99–100) there are at least four such functions:

1. Communication plays an indispensable part in relationships between practitioners and clients, as it does in all relationships between people. As well as its more general functions, there are particularly important issues with regard to information and consent.

2. Communication provides a way of *informing the patient* about the nature and likely course of his or her condition and the therapeutic manoeuvres possible, in order to secure appropriate informed consent to further diagnostic and therapeutic measures (Gafni et al. 1998).
3. Communication is a means to assist patients in understanding the intended treatments and decisions that may be taken. This will not only attain informed consent, but also may enhance concordance between patient and practitioner concerning the agreed-upon treatments.
4. Most importantly, says Widder (2004), communication allows us to attain knowledge about the symptoms and their personal relevance to the patient, so that the diagnostic process can be appropriately targeted and so we can find out what is at stake for the patient as a person.

There are several implications here which are worth pausing over. First, it means that in order to understand communication in health care contexts we must grasp the culture of the people interacting. Ways of expressing pain, displaying knowledge and deference, talking to colleagues, speaking to health care practitioners about the symptoms of a partner or child and so on, are all given shape, form and meaning through culture. How we 'do' or perform these activities depends on our 'habitus' as described in Chapter 1, and our intuitive grasp of the 'doxa' or rules of the game.

It is also a fundamental assumption of these approaches that communication is a primordial element of the health care process and is basic to the health care encounter. Thus, communication is not merely an accidental event that could eventually be supplanted by some other diagnostic technique: it is, says Widder (2004), a *necessary and irreplaceable* part of the process of attaining essential medical knowledge. In Widder's view communicative events presuppose two subjects: the subject expressing their experiences and the subject who is attempting to understand these experiences. In many cases these understandings are brought together with biomedical, psychosocial or other causal theories about disease. This kind of knowledge may in the first place be difficult to reconcile with the tenets of evidence-based practice if we take them in a strong form. However, it leads to a shared understanding between practitioner and client about what is at stake for the client. For practitioners, the knowledge they gain this way forms the basis of their potential to practise the art and science of health care, and act in the patient's interest, as it is in this way that health care can be based on the patient's experiences and evaluations that make up the phenomenon and phenomenology of disease. Indeed, as Sarangi (2004) indicates in his influential editorial launching the new journal, *Communication and Medicine*, the last 30 years have seen a profound growth in the study of health care encounters and interaction, and consequently the visibility of such research to health care professionals has been enhanced.

Within this often interdisciplinary research movement a number of hints are emerging in the literature about the importance and power of communication. It is by communicating effectively about the client's circumstances and competing concerns that a satisfactory outcome can be achieved.

To take an example, new mothers have many contacts with primary health care providers such as GPs and maternal and child health nurses, yet many problems are not disclosed; only 1 in 3 women experiencing depression will seek help, and physical problems often go unreported (Gunn et al. 2003). In fields as diverse as continence care (Shaw et al. 2000), maternity care (Rowe et al. 2002), infant death (Rowe et al. 2001) and heart surgery (Davies 2000) there appears to be an under-reporting of distress and pain, which appears to be associated with subsequent dissatisfaction with services. There may even be cases where patients desperate for treatment which they believe will bring them relief use a variety of communicative strategies to convince doctors to perform operations on them, such as hysterectomies (Salmon and Marchant-Haycox 2000). Persuasion, presenting evidence and arguments in a convincing way and even outright manipulation may occur on both sides of the consulting room desk.

More generally, the giving and receiving of stories has a significant place in health care activity. As Enkin and Jadad (1998: 963) remind us, 'Anecdotes are powerful tools that humans use to make decisions'. Whereas the role of storytelling in psychotherapy has recently been explored (Crawford et al. 2004), there are as yet few attempts to reconcile storytelling approaches elsewhere in the health care process with the ambitions of the evidence-based movement. This is an issue to which we shall return later in the chapter as we describe some of the critiques which have been mounted of a strong evidence-based approach in health communication. In a sense, stories, narratives and other verbal performances are a kind of 'practice-based evidence' that we ignore at our peril.

The evidence of practice: room for improvement

The last 20 years have seen a growing sense that health care professionals are tending to communicate less effectively or warmly with their clients. Observers of the scenes in hospitals and clinics returned reports like the following:

> In the settings I observed ... the main reason for patient contact was to obtain information for medical charts. To accomplish this primary objective while restricting other demands of their heavy case loads, the interns and residents collectively developed several strategies: (1) avoiding patients and their families; (2) narrowing the focus of interaction to strictly 'medical' concerns; and (3) treating patients as non-persons – even in their presence. They used medical terminology which was incomprehensible to most patients and often looked past them, avoiding eye contact. Patients, and, especially, family members, were frequently treated as if they were invisible.
>
> (Mizrahi 1984: 160)

Two decades after this it was as if little had changed. At the time of writing, a National Audit Office (2005: 47) report on patient safety in the National Health Service states that 'Complaints are mainly about: poor communication with patients and relatives, poor clinical practice, unsatisfactory patient experience, poor staff attitude and poor complaints handling'.

Moreover the 'adverse incidents' in health care where patients' wellbeing is harmed through accident and error were frequently blamed on 'poor communication'. 'Communication failure' was named among the top five problems leading to adverse incidents. Hence there is increasing emphasis on getting staff to communicate in such a way as to minimize risk. 'In future junior doctors will have to demonstrate their competence in communication and consultation skills' as the National Audit Office (2005: 17) counsels gravely.

Priest et al. (2005) note that communication is an area of practice where practitioners often fail to satisfy clients, and poor communication between different groups of health care professionals, with clients and with carers, is a frequent cause of grievance and litigation (Health Service Ombudsman for England 2003). Furthermore, the quality of communication between different professional groups affects health care outcomes, and failures in this regard have contributed to the tragedies that have been the subject of national inquiries in the UK. For example, let us consider the Bristol Royal Infirmary Inquiry (2001) into concerns over the high mortality rate associated with operations on children's hearts. Here it was concluded that communication between some staff and parents was poor and there did not appear to have been any serious thinking about the way that information was communicated to parents and the young patients before operations. Staff improvised and apparently drew helpful diagrams, sometimes on discarded paper towels. Yet as the Inquiry team note, often the issue of getting consent from parents and patients was seen as a chore. 'Good communication is essential, but as the Royal College of Surgeons of England told us: ". . . it is the area of greatest compromise in the practices of most surgeons in the NHS and the source of most complaints" (Bristol Royal Infirmary Inquiry 2001: 13)'. Now, a diagram drawn on a scrap of paper is not necessarily inferior to a slick PowerPoint display or video whose production was sponsored by a pharmaceutical company. The latter do not necessarily imply better communication, and a little impromptu diagram drawing has at least a sense of sincerity and desire to tailor the presentation to the client's needs. However, the point is that communication had not been factored into the process, and was secondary to the desire to undertake operations.

Despite the widespread belief that failures of communication can be catastrophic, Priest et al. (2005) point to the fact that, as they see it, there is as yet little research into the effectiveness of communication skills training in health care. The UK's Department of Health (2003) clearly wants health practitioners to be appropriately skilled at the point of professional registration. The Department of Health is also keen to acknowledge the scope for education providers to work together to share learning materials, innovations and good practice relating to communication skills. Yet despite this enthusiasm and the proliferation of research on the subject of communication, it is sometimes surprising how little has changed as a result of all these efforts. Let us explore a little more in the next section of what is known about the way that practitioners communicate with one another – an under-researched area despite its acknowledged importance in helping to ensure quality of care and avert tragedies.

So, despite several decades of communication skills training, the issues remain stubbornly prominent. 'Poor communication' is still blamed for accidents, failures, patient dissatisfaction, complaints and litigation. Yet we still do not seem to be able to offer recommendations that unequivocally help in these situations.

Communication: skills, evidence and everyday communicative practice

Maybe we are trying to make sense of the issue in the wrong way. As Skelton and Hobbs (1999: 578) remark, communication is often thought of as a skill, and that doing it well were a matter of rehearsing discrete pieces of surface behaviour. Communication can be fostered by 'an atmosphere of empathy' and this seems to be associated with 'clusters of cooperative language'. However, we cannot easily imagine how this kind of clustering could be formally taught so that students could learn it and reliably reproduce it. Skelton (2005) later proposes that the skills are only part of the story. When they are written down, they can seem banal or even trivial – being polite to the patient, involving them in decision making, allowing them to feel that they are being listened to, and so on. A good practitioner, however, can command a variety of skills and use them appropriately and they are underpinned by understanding the context of the encounter, attitudes to clients, to medicine and professional life itself. This, he suggests, is much more difficult to teach and learn.

Thus whereas there are desirable features of the health care encounter which educators want trainee health professionals to learn, even experienced medical educators find that there are some aspects which are very difficult to include in this framework.

The pervasive evidence–practice gap in health care which has concerned so many authors (Whitstock 2003) may be gradually closed by means of efforts of this kind. But the difficulty may also be partly attributed to the nature of the scientific undertaking itself. The process of drawing inferences from clinical studies is 'not only a question of statistical generalization, but must include a jump from the world of experience into the world of reason, assessment and theoretical judgment' (Holmberg et al. 1999: 160). In addition, it may be difficult for clinicians and researchers to fully grasp what a medical condition means to the client. Evidence of the significance of diseases and interventions from the patient's perspective is less clearly defined in the research literature, despite a decade or so of research on illness narratives (Widder 2004). Thus there are areas where more evidence may still be needed, even on well-researched topics, and we may still need to organize data and insights more effectively so that the implications for clinical practice can be readily apprehended.

Many authors have now grasped the importance of assimilating evidence into everyday communicative practice in health care (Bradley and Humphreys 1999) but how this should be achieved is far less clear. Equally, there is some uncertainty as to how to incorporate evidence about effective communication strategies into clinical training. In the face of this uncertainty, some attempts have so far been made, for example by Roter et al. (2004), who have explored the use of video training programmes to facilitate the development of skills such as listening to clients and a reduction in clinicians' verbal dominance, increased use of open-ended questions, increased use of empathy, and increased partnership building and problem solving for therapeutic regimen.

This usefully shows a pathway to encourage desirable features of communication. Some authors go further and have sought to enhance the autonomy and ability of clients to make evidence-based choices themselves (Walter et al. 2004).

Communication between practitioners

As well as the encounter between client and practitioner, the evidence-based approach to health care communication has important implications for communication between practitioners. Communication between professional groups has long been acknowledged to be problematic. There are complaints and concerns that methods of transferring information are inadequate and that this leads to poor uptake of services, dissatisfaction for workers, and poorer patient outcomes (Payne et al. 2002). Equally, there are a number of simple strategies which have been demonstrated to improve situations like this. The use of written information to accompany the transitions between different phases of care such as going from intensive care to a general ward (Paul et al. 2004) has been found to be beneficial.

Practitioners frequently complain about the difficulties which stem from having to communicate with other groups of professionals and teams in other institutions. Cornbleet et al. (2002) reported that there was a widespread belief in primary care teams that information from hospitals takes too long to reach them, leading to difficulties and delays in offering support and advice to clients. This is particularly apparent when the patient's problems are most severe. In the case of what they call 'malignant disease', the patient's 'journey' can often involve many clinical teams distributed through several hospitals. In the management of cancer, patients may encounter a very large number of practitioners (Smith et al. 1999). In order to overcome the problems relating to the transfer of information the use of patient-held records has been established in a number of disciplines. That way, the records arrive with the patients, provided they have not forgotten them or left them on a bus. In obstetrics (Lovell et al. 1987), child health (Macfarlane 1992) and chronic illness (Essex et al. 1990) patient-held records have been used so as to avoid duplication and as part of a move towards greater patient involvement in decision making. In cancer care, studies have suggested that this is welcomed by patients but is sometimes difficult to introduce (Finlay and Watt 1999). Making patients themselves the vehicle for the transmission of information can aid timely, problem-focused care. Yet even this brings with it some disadvantages. Practitioners will very likely spend some of the all-too-frequently brief consultation frantically skimming through the records, occasionally glancing up to look at the patient over the top of their glasses. This situation then is often scarcely any less satisfactory, and brings us on to the crucial question of how practitioners communicate with clients.

Communication between practitioners and clients

As educators, practitioners, and professional and statutory bodies around the world are increasingly recognizing, communication is a core clinical skill for practitioners. As Fallowfield et al. (2002) note, in the course of a 40-year career, a hospital doctor might undertake around 150,000 to 200,000 consultations with patients and their families. However, despite recent changes in training for student practitioners in many health care disciplines, very few of the older generation of doctors in practice have received much formal training in communication, and the training provided would be thought inadequate by contemporary standards. According to research carried out in the 1990s (Fallowfield 1995; Ramirez et al. 1995) senior doctors recognize that their difficulties in this area contribute to high psychological morbidity, emotional burnout, depersonalization, and low sense of personal accomplishment.

Equally, there are many insights from the literature and personal experience that communicative aspects of care are the source of much dissatisfaction for clients too. For example, here is a mother talking about nursing advice for a crying colicky baby:

> You get a little disappointed because you don't hear anything new (at the child health centre). We are constantly looking for something that might help, if there is anything we can do to make her feel better. And the mass of tips you get (from the nurse), you have just heard them thousands of times before and you have tried them all and nothing really helps.
>
> (Helseth 2002: 270)

In the same study, here is a father talking about what could be gained from the experience of interacting with the staff:

> If I could meet a person who was involved in what I said, even if she didn't have much advice to give, but tried to lift me up to a level where I felt I got help, and that we got a little feedback on the things we were struggling with as parents, then I am sure I would be on a quite different level when leaving the clinic, and have more mental strength to get on with my work, the work of being a father.
>
> (p. 271)

Thus, even when the semantic content of the advice does not necessarily offer anything more than what is known already, it is the quality of the communication which yields the sense that one is being helped. From studies like these it is clear that clients and patients can be remarkably forgiving when health care staff do not have anything concrete to offer, but it is their sense that the practitioner is 'involved' in what they say or that they are being listened to.

Even when therapeutic regimes themselves are built upon the best available evidence, there may still be sources of disquiet. Feltham (2005: 136) suggested that certain individuals who have had the most meticulously evidence-based cognitive therapy for anxiety and depression subsequently did not feel they had benefited. They felt they had not been understood and listened to as unique individuals; instead therapists were intent on following through their rather stilted, manual-like strategies.

In addition, it is sometimes difficult to get practitioners themselves to take the value of communication skills, and most particularly the practice of being trained in them, seriously. Feinmann (2002: 1572) comments that 'of all the pressing concerns facing doctors today, taking lessons in talking to patients is way down the list'. Former consultant, Evan Harris, speaking in his role as a member of parliament for the Liberal Democrat Party, was reported as saying, 'I would query whether people who spend their working lives communicating need classes run by psychologists', when asked to comment on proposals to further develop communication skills in UK doctors' training.

Feinmann (2002) also notes that surgeons are often among the most resistant to 'acknowledg[e] the need to brush up their talking skills'. Nevertheless, the UK's Royal College of Surgeons is treating this as a cause for concern. As the then chair of the patient liaison group, Charles Collins, remarked, 'We tend to go into training because we like the technical aspects. Yet only around 25 per cent of the surgeon's job requires technical expertise, even less in many specialities. The rest is about communicating with patients' (Feinmann 2002: 1572).

Even in surgery then communication is the royal pathway to patient-centred medicine. Hence, the key in strengthening the evidence-base of patient-centred medicine is to be found in communication research. Much important work is already done in the field of communication in health care. Through the research completed so far, there are some important insights into the kind of communication behaviour which is most effective in health care consultations in general. For instance the relevance of affective behaviour, especially nonverbal behaviour, is well documented in creating a positive impression for both client and practitioner (DiMatteo et al. 1986; Bensing et al. 1996). There is a growing amount of evidence on gender issues in medical communication (Bensing et al. 1993); effect studies on training programmes have given evidence on what communication behaviours can be taught and trained (Anderson and Sharpe 1991; Levinson and Roter 1993; Roter et al. 1995; Smith et al. 1998).

Evidence in practice: the power of anecdotes and clients' preferences

The experience of evidence in practice usually starts not from a scientific account of research, but from the kinds of stories told by clients to professionals. These might be tragic, moving or affecting, as well as trivial, sublime or ridiculous. Evidence in practice, or practice-based evidence (Fox, 2003) is often grounded in stories. As we noted earlier, Enkin and Jadad (1998) remind us that anecdotes are powerful tools that humans use to make decisions. Bleakley (2005) describes the ways in which narrative and storytelling can add to the more conventionally rigorous inquiries favoured within health care. As he remarks, qualitative studies have often been seen as 'soft', in contrast to the 'hard' sciences. Indeed, as Gherardi and Turner (2002) put it, 'real men don't collect soft data'. However, narrative enquiry's supposedly soft data can illuminate hard realities. For example, in a study devoted to the impact of trauma surgery on 48 young black survivors of 'penetrating violence', Rich and Grey (2003) employed in-depth interviews which elicited narrative accounts that yielded dramatic insight into the fear of death, the lives of these socially marginalized patients, and the important role of health care personnel in transforming these experiences for the better. Moreover, it seemed that participants were empowered as a result of the researchers showing an interest in their worlds. As Bleakley (2005) remarks, while numerical morbidity and mortality data are usually 'faceless', narrative enquiry by contrast often seeks to personalize and to engage proactively with its research participants who become valued informants and co-researchers who explore the experience collaboratively with the investigators.

The role of sympathetic attention in formulating good relations between patients and practitioners and in leading to favourably judged outcomes has been documented elsewhere. In cancer care Fallowfield and Jenkins (2004) note that there is an emerging consensus about how patients want to be told news about their illness and what they need to hear. The desire for an empathic delivery was reported by Girgis et al. (1999) where patients with breast cancer said they wanted the diagnosis and prognosis to be given in simple language; honestly, but not too bluntly. In a study by Friedrichsen et al. (2002) in Sweden, patients interpreted information conveyed to them about ending active tumour treatment as either emotionally trying or as fortifying and strengthening. This appeared to relate to the way that words used had focused the patients' attention on either treatment, quality of life issues, or towards threat and death. Summarizing the information provided to patients with cancer can assist their understanding and lead to their adhering to treatment recommendations or advice more fully, and enables them to make more informed decisions about possible treatment options.

Thus, even at the heart of evidence-based communication for practitioners and clients, where the preferences of clients and the outcomes of encounters are meticulously researched, the kinds of narratives which are co-constructed by clients and practitioners are vitally important.

The role of narratives on the part of both the client and practitioner is by no means clear cut, however. There may be elements which involve both parties in dilemmas. For example, in dealing with bad news for patients, many practitioners express uncertainty about 'getting the balance right' (Fallowfield and Jenkins 2004). This involves the value of being honest but at the same time the need to be encouraging, hopeful and supportive. This is illustrated in a study by Kim and Alvi (1999) of experiences of patients with head and neck cancer. Patients wanted their doctors to be 'truthful, caring, and compassionate', to speak in simple terms, and to use unambiguous language. In cancer consultations ambiguity is commonplace, perhaps because euphemistic expressions are commonly used to 'soften the blow'. However, this means that health professionals can convey an unintended meaning without being aware that they have done so.

These dilemmas and difficulties with communication may result in disjunctures between the understanding held by the professional and that of the client. For example, in some studies it appeared that patients with advanced malignant disease were unaware of their diagnosis and outlook (Chan and Woodruff 1997). A corollary of this is that they might misunderstand the therapeutic intent of treatment (Quirt et al. 1997). Some terms, like 'positive' and 'negative nodes', and phrases like 'the disease is progressing' may have different connotations when used in a clinical rather than a lay context and might alarm or falsely reassure patients in a manner which is difficult for the clinician to predict (Chapman et al. 2003).

The degree of alignment between clinicians' and patients' views of what the important issues are in a clinical encounter can also be influenced by the kinds of questions asked. Fallowfield et al. (2002) advise against using too many leading questions in the collection of clinical information so as to yield more accurate data collection, in the hope that this can lead to better management decisions. Fallowfield and colleagues recommend the use of open then focused questions so as to enable more dialogue with the patient, which also is believed to lead to more efficient data gathering about symptoms. The use of a more open style of questioning can yield important gains in information when side-effects and other unanticipated symptoms are being discussed. Clinicians' impressions about side-effects may be very different from patients' own experiences, perhaps because clinicians have relied on closed questioning (Fellowes et al. 2001). A more open-ended questioning style also yields a greater sense of empathy, which may encourage a better doctor–patient relationship, allowing the patient to feel more valued and consequently more comfortable about disclosing potentially sensitive information.

Here, it can be seen that attention to clients' preferences with particular illnesses in specific cultures can yield more effective ways of communicating, allowing greater acquisition of information and a greater sense on the part of clients that they are being listened to and treated with respect. The story of communication in life-threatening situations as told by Bleakley, Fallowfield and their colleagues is one where clients and physicians have worked together to achieve greater understanding with consequent benefits to both.

This dialectical and dilemmatic relationship between professionals and clients can involve other intriguing aspects. The relationship between professionals and patients is often dialectical in the sense that it is an integral whole where the participants are mutually interdependent. For example, Salmon and Marchant-Haycox (2000) were intrigued by the possibility that patients might try to influence their doctor's decision. In some cases, patients appear to have been able to convince the doctors to undertake an operation such as a hysterectomy in the absence of any obvious physical pathology. Indeed, some of the gynaecologists involved in the study perceived the patients as influential too, especially those who were more apt to describe the social effects of the symptoms, to catastrophize, and specifically to request a hysterectomy. As the authors conclude, this may merely be a part of the process and a good deal of influence may take place of which the physician is not fully aware. Clients who have imbued themselves with the milieu and spirit of health care can perhaps develop such an expertise that they are able to ensure that things turn out to their advantage.

Thus, an ability to embed oneself within culture and display the appropriate symptoms to a suitable degree of authenticity is crucial to getting the operation one wants. Moreover, it shows that there are powerful expectations held by some participants. If one imagines the nature of hysterectomies, with the potentially hazardous, painful and debilitating surgery involved, one must need to be very convinced as to the potential benefits in order to press ahead with it and try so hard to convince one's doctor. Here again, the role of culture, and background knowledge of attitudes and beliefs about the anatomical insignia of femininity is crucial. The issue of habitus – those aspects of culture that are anchored in the body or daily practices of individuals, groups and societies – is a vital part of the process. This is not to say that patients who desire operations are in any way deliberately faking. It is more that culture provides the spaces into which their distress can unfold. According to sociological theorists such as Norbert Elias (1969) and Marcel Mauss (1990) habitus includes the totality of learned habits, bodily skills, styles, tastes, and other non-discursive knowledges that might be said to 'go without saying' for a specific group. Thus in a fundamental sense, we know how to be ill, as if it were natural. This was brought home to one of us (BB) while in hospital with kidney stones. Whereas the majority of the people on the ward were bearing their suffering stoically, including those with a myriad of brightly coloured tubes sprouting from their pyjamas, the relative quiet of the situation was interrupted by the admission of an elderly Polish man. He was lamenting volubly. Indeed, so vocal was he that he was eventually taken away to another part of the hospital, but his lamenting and keening could still be heard echoing along the corridors. This man's response might point to marked differences in the way that distress is 'naturally' presented, and the way that health care personnel 'naturally' respond even within the apparently homogeneous cultural landscape of Europe.

Theories of communication and theories of disease

Communication is partly about the mechanics of interaction but it reflects considerably more. The question of evidence and its relation to communicative behaviour can run much deeper than this. The way that people communicate and what they communicate about reflect the kinds of informal and implicit theories they may have about the nature of the problem. These furthermore reflect a whole range of half-submerged assumptions and beliefs about the nature of disease and the roles of sufferers and healers, the demeanour of illness and the conduct of a helping professional. They stretch out to intersect with wider patterns of common sense and common culture. Thus, the communication strategies adopted by health care professionals may recollect in miniature some of the major theories about the causes of disease and disorder. An acquaintance of one of the authors who is an osteopath says he tends to wear a white coat on his first encounter with a new 'patient' because 'it looks more professional' yet reverts to more informal dress on subsequent occasions once a therapeutic relationship has been achieved. This is particularly interesting in the light of the recent history of osteopathy, which has often had to struggle for acceptance in the health care world. Adopting medical insignia such as a white coat has important connotations in these circumstances. Or to take another example, understanding human distress in terms of a biomedical framework can leave a practitioner impatient with psychosocial matters, worries and dilemmas, and keen instead to carve through to what he or she thinks of as the root of the matter.

Changing practitioners' world views and their theoretical understanding of human problems might well make them more favourably disposed towards conversations about psychological, familial and social matters with their clients. Gunn et al. (2003) describe a programme of education in interviewing skills for general practitioners (GPs) in working with clients who had recently had babies. The programme successfully enhanced the elicitation of information about postnatal problems through the practice of active listening skills and the ability to identify cues in the consultation that merited further enquiry by the practitioner. This programme went further and challenged practitioners through the introduction of evidence that questioned some of their firmly held beliefs. Around half the GPs expressed surprise that evidence was lacking for a hormonal basis of maternal depression and that psychological and drug therapies were equally effective management strategies. Between a third and half of these GPs were willing to accept the evidence and change their minds.

This kind of enquiry suggests that health practitioners will be more inclined to attend to those parts of the problem which they believe to be theoretically important and practically significant. It is commonly complained that physicians, psychiatrists and to some extent nurses too, undertake a training which tends to emphasize biological aspects of disease as primary rather than expanding their point of view to consider psychological, social and economic factors that might have been crucial in bringing the client to the clinic. However, returning to the issues which we addressed in the first chapter, the kind of local culture, or habitus if you will, of medicine, tends to predispose an interest in the physical aspects of the human condition and a concomitant belief that its mysteries will one day be found in the flesh. When dealing with complex human problems however, this can lead to a relatively narrow focus. Moreover it can be associated with a tendency to see the mosaic of problems as indicating a particular pathogenic theory. For example, to take the currently widespread condition of childhood, attention deficit hyperactivity disorder (ADHD), there is considerable scepticism in methodological terms concerning research which claims to show differences in the brains of children with ADHD and those without. The children with ADHD in such studies are almost always ones with considerable exposure to Ritalin or other stimulant drugs (Leo and Cohen 2003) and researchers do not report comparisons between medication-naïve and medicated children (Cohen and Leo 2004) who in any case also often differ in terms of age, body size and other variables. This level of methodological detail is missing from 'consensus statements' on the subject such as that by Barkley et al. (2002). However, thinking about the assumptions and expectations that might be encouraged in health professionals reading the literature, it is easy to see how they might privilege the physical aspects of the syndrome rather than social or communicative aspects. The way the debate is foreclosed and information is structured encourages a particular kind of communication.

Moreover, an evidence-based approach to health care more generally can stimulate curiosity and attentiveness on the part of practitioners, even if the available evidence relates largely to physical aspects of patients' conditions. Practitioners with enquiring minds might find it challenging, stimulating and also fun to see if each new person offers fresh challenges for the existing theories to explain or encourages us to think anew about the conventional wisdom in the discipline.

It might also be possible to stimulate scientific and evidence-based curiosity concerning the communicative process itself. Feinmann (2002: 1572) quotes Lucille Ong of Amsterdam's Academic Medical Centre: 'Doctors become enthusiastic when confronted with their own consultation style and receiving feedback from a professional, encouraging them to practice "difficult consultations" in role play'.

The stimulation of this curiosity might go even further. It might yield the application of a critical intelligence to the idea of evidence-based practice itself. We have seen how some students of health care communication have tried to identify the mutual lines of influence between practitioner and client, and how this process may be seen as a dialectical one – that is, one that moves to resolve contradictory ideas or arguments and brings into focus the full range of changes and interactions that occur in the world (Ollman 2003). In the next section then we shall take this dialectical approach a little further and describe some of the debates and critiques of evidence-based practice in health care a little more fully so as to show these dialectical processes at work.

The critique of evidence-based practice revisited: the possibilities for practice-based evidence

The difficulties in reconciling communicative activity in health care with the spirit of evidence-based medicine are compounded by the fact that as communication becomes more complex and two-directional – indeed dialectical in its own right – it becomes more difficult to measure. Generally, the drift of the existing evidence is that more communication is a good thing, and that the more it resembles friendly conversation the greater the payoff in terms of client satisfaction. Yet the more it sounds like a conversational dialogue the more difficult it is to reduce it to a manual or protocol, the more difficult it is to measure and evaluate. This is even more problematic when it involves a whole group of people such as we might find involved in family therapy, or team-based care. Larner (2004) outlines a number of concerns about family therapy in this regard but they could equally well apply anywhere where clients and their families are involved in a complex dialogue with health or social care professionals. Therapists may apply techniques flexibly and pragmatically in response to the perceived needs of the client in contexts. This becomes even more difficult to quantify given the growing popularity of integrative models in social care, psychotherapy and family therapy.

There is also an implicit understanding in a good deal of the evidence-based literature that health care is about applying some sort of intervention, whether this be surgical, pharmacological or communicative, and trying to identify the effects. However, in some therapies, especially those of a more reflective cast, the role of therapy might be more to highlight personal and systemic narratives, and encourage families and individuals to reflect upon their stories. Therapists may even step back from specific interventions. In other words, says Larner (2004), therapies may best be seen as ecological interventions in peoples' natural environments that do not easily translate into a step-by-step procedure or the kind of intervention that can be itemized in a manual so as to be repeatedly applied and tested.

There is a concern among many researchers and practitioners that evidence-based practice represents a kind of deprofessionalization. As Jordan and Jordan (2000: 209) say: 'Evidence-based care would be a very good way to tie the profession … into a conception of their tasks that effectively deskilled and shackled them, while seeming to raise their status to that of scientific researchers'.

Yet the basis upon which this apparent deskilling is taking place is itself questioned by some authors. Bensing (2000) notes, for example, that randomized controlled trials are performed on diseases, while the results have to be applied to patients that in many cases would not have fulfilled the inclusion criteria for participation in the study.

Physicians and other health professionals can experience a sense of tension between their roles as scientists and their roles as care givers. This is movingly described by Cassell in *The Nature of Suffering and the Goals of Medicine* (1991). Enhancing the extent to which evidence-based health care can be patient-centred, perhaps by incorporating patients' views into randomized controlled trials, may benefit patients, but also diminish the tension that is felt by physicians in their double role as scientist and carer.

Taking the idea of transformation and critique of evidence-based approaches a little further, we can identify a number of opposing positions which offer alternatives to a strong evidence-based approach. These often start from a position which is sceptical of the modernist conception of knowledge and the grand narrative of scientific progress with which it is often aligned. As Fox (2003) reminds us, many post-Enlightenment theories of knowledge have an implicit agenda which assumes, in the manner of the popular 1990s science fiction TV series *The X Files* that 'the truth is out there'. They dress it up in various ways, for example in terms of concerns with validity and reliability, or perhaps in the case of qualitative research, in terms of authenticity or credibility. However, over the past few decades there have been many thinkers loosely clustering around post-modernist or post-structuralist viewpoints who have voiced an increasing suspicion of these kinds of 'grand narratives' or attempts to develop accounts of the 'truth' in a verifiable, finalized way. The concern with science, truth and rationality in modernism has been undermined by radical scepticism in post-modernism. The post-modern spirit then is one of suspicion of 'grand narratives' that purport to offer a unified or veridically truthful perspective on the world. Derrida (1976) describes these kinds of narratives, for example, philosophy, theology, science, biomedicine or historical studies, as *logocentrisms*, whose objective is to achieve the *logos* – unmediated truth about the world. As Fox (2003) points out, there are many examples of apparently excellent science that have not yielded the hoped-for innovations in practice because researchers and practitioners hold different priorities and agendas. Furthermore, even in countries which nominally subscribe to scientific medicine, practice can vary widely (Sweeney and Kernick 2002), for example in cardiothoracic surgery between Britain and the USA (Brook et al. 1988), and in prescription patterns in different European countries (Garratini and Garratini 1993).

As a way of dealing with these kinds of phenomena, which would be problematic from the point of view of asserting a single right way of doing things, Fox (2003) proposes instead 'practice-based evidence', a different kind of relationship between research and practice. He advocates that first, the pursuit of knowledge should be seen as a local and contingent process, rather than seeking grand generalizations. Second, he says that research activity should take a proactive stance towards differences, and rather than classify or place phenomena in a hierarchy research should question whether certain forms of knowing are legitimated at the expense of knowledge as a whole. We should perhaps ask: whose interests does knowledge serve? Finally, says Fox, it would be desirable to see theory building as an adjunct to practical activity, and evaluate it in terms of its ability to make a practical contribution to the setting where it originated. Together, these recommendations would help to dissolve the oppositions between the researcher and those being researched and the divide between research and practice. Fox desires to see ethically and politically engaged research that can contribute to practice-based evidence as well as evidence-based practice.

A further limitation on whether evidence-based practice can characterize what happens in health care encounters is to do with the nature of knowledge. The practical approach in much health care still bears the imprint of 'see one, do one, teach one'. As if knowledge could be acquired through observation and practice and then taught by the experienced practitioner to the novice. Yet there may be inherent restrictions on this process. According to Polanyi (1983), human knowing involves us knowing more than we can impart. A person might have comprehensive knowledge manifested through their ability to perform complicated actions, for example communicating flawlessly, yet at the same time they may be unable to explain their actions. In health care settings Polanyi identifies the practice of diagnosis as involving expert observation and skilful testing, which is often difficult to describe explicitly. If Polanyi is correct then this makes it difficult to itemize and characterize the kinds of skills we are aiming to promote. Instead they lie in those half-implicit areas of practice that we described as part of the 'habitus' or 'doxa' in Chapter 1.

Schön (1991) describes the ability of experienced practitioners to consider what they know intuitively in the midst of action as 'reflection-in-action'. Reflection-in-action is seen as a sort of unconscious and inarticulate 'conversation with the situation', where reframing and reworking of the problem leads to it being restructured and hence solved. The practitioner's absorption in the culture of the health care setting and their repertoire of examples, images, understandings and actions enable their capacity for dealing with unique situations and individuals. This practical, clinical knowledge is gradually developed as the practitioner gains in experience. In clinical work, tacit knowing concerning the nature of the problems encountered, and a tacit knowledge of the rules of the institutional and professional game – the 'doxa' – constitute important parts of diagnostic reasoning and judgment. Experienced practitioners apply a range of experiential knowledge and strategies that are part of this habitus in Bourdieu's sense of the term, which are hardly mentioned in the textbooks. Critical analysis of data is a key skill for students and clinicians to master, although there is evidence that the level of skill may be suboptimal (Stern et al. 1995).

Conclusion

The message from much of what we have reviewed here is that as well as 'skills' of the kind that are inculcated in communication training where practitioners are urged to use more eye contact or ask more open questions, what is also needed is motivational and cultural change. Health care teams have to feel that communication with patients is a good idea and be committed to it, whereupon the warmth and enthusiasm may well be more effective than the specific collection of techniques employed. As such there is a clear need to shift the search for evidence beyond identifying and validating elementary components of effective communication towards knowing how professionals in real clinical places can be contracted to good communication performance. In other words, it is not that we require evidence to underpin communication approaches so urgently as evidence of promoting factors in good communication practices. Yet to date there is little knowledge surrounding this.

References

Anderson, L.A. and Sharpe, P.A. (1991) Improving patient and provider communication: a synthesis and review of communication interventions, *Patient Education and Counselling*, 17: 99–134.

Audit Commission (1996) *Misspent Youth*. London: Audit Commission.

Barkley, R., Cook, E., Diamond, A. et al. (2002) International consensus statement on ADHD, *Clinical Child and Family Psychology Review*, 5: 89–111.

Bensing, J. (2000) Bridging the gap: the separate worlds of evidence-based medicine and patient-centered medicine, *Patient Education and Counseling*, 39: 17–25.

Bensing, J.M., van den Brink-Muinen, A. and Bakker, D.H. (1993) Gender differences in practice style: a Dutch study of general practitioners, *Medical Care*, 31: 219–29.

Bensing, J.M., Schreurs, K.M.G. and De Rijk A. (1996) The role of the general practitioner's affective behaviour in medical encounters, *Psychology of Health*, 11: 825–38.

Bleakley, A. (2005) Stories as data, data as stories: making sense of narrative inquiry in clinical education, *Medical Education,* 39: 534–40.

Bradley, P. and Humphreys, G. (1999) Assessing the ability of medical students to apply evidence in practice: the potential of the OSCE, *Medical Education*, 33 815–17.

Bristol Royal Infirmary Inquiry (2001) *Learning from Bristol: The Report of the Public Inquiry into Children's Heart Surgery at the Bristol Royal Infirmary 1984–1995*. London: Stationery Office, Cm 5207 (1).

Brook, R.H., Park R.E. and Winslow C.M. (1988) Diagnosis and treatment of coronary disease: a comparison of doctors' attitudes in the USA and the UK, *Lancet*, 189: 7550–3.

Brown, B., Crawford, P. and Hicks, C. (2003) *Evidence-based Research: Dilemmas and Debates in Health Care*. Buckingham: Open University Press.

Cassell, E. (1991) *The Nature of Suffering and the Goals of Medicine*. New York: Oxford University Press.

Chan, A. and Woodruff, R.K. (1997) Communicating with patients with advanced cancer, *Journal of Palliative Care*, 13: 29–33.

Chapman, K., Abraham, C., Jenkins, V. and Fallowfield, L. (2003) Lay understanding of terms used in cancer consultations, *Psycho-oncology*, 12: 557–66.

Cohen, D. and Leo, J. (2004) An update on ADHD neuroimaging research, *Journal of Mind and Behavior*, 25(2): 161–6.

Cornbleet, M.A., Campbell, P. Murray, S., Stevenson, M. and Bond, S. (2002) Patient-held records in cancer and palliative care: a randomized, prospective trial, *Palliative Medicine*, 16: 205–12.

Crawford, P., Brown, B., Anthony, P. and Hicks, C. (2002) Reluctant empiricists: community mental health nurses and the art of evidence-based praxis, *Health and Social Care in the Community*, 10(4): 287–98.

Crawford, R., Brown, B. and Crawford, P. (2004) *Storytelling in Therapy*. Cheltenham: Nelson Thornes.

Davies, N. (2000) Patients' and carers' perceptions of factors influencing recovery after cardiac surgery, *Journal of Advanced Nursing*, 32(2): 318–26.

Department of Health (1996) *Promoting Clinical Effectiveness: A Framework for Action in and through the NHS*. London: Department of Health.

Department of Health (2003) *Guiding Principles Relating to the Commissioning and Provision of Communication Skills Training in Pre-registration and Undergraduate Education for Healthcare Professionals.* Leeds: Department of Health.

Derrida, J. (1976) *Of Grammatology.* Baltimore, MD: Johns Hopkins University Press.

DiMatteo, M.R., Hays, R.D. and Prince, L.M. (1986) Relationship of physicians' nonverbal communication skill to patient satisfaction, appointment noncompliance, and physician workload, *Health Psychology,* 5: 581–94.

Economic and Social Research Council (ESRC) (2001) *Programme on Research Method.* London: ESRC.

Elias, N. (1969) *The Civilizing Process, Volume I. The History of Manners.* Oxford: Blackwell.

Enkin, M.W. and Jadad, A.R. (1998) Using anecdotal information in evidence-based health care: heresy or necessity? *Annals of Oncology,* 9: 963–6.

Essex, B., Doig, R. and Renshaw, J. (1990) Pilot study of records of shared care for people with mental illness, *British Medical Journal,* 300: 1442–6.

Evidence-based Medicine Working Group (1992) Evidence-based medicine: a new approach to teaching the practice of medicine, *Journal of the American Medical Association,* 268: 2420–5.

Fallowfield, L.J. (1995) Can we improve the professional and personal fulfillment of doctors in cancer medicine? *British Journal of Cancer,* 71: 1132–3.

Fallowfield, L.J. and Jenkins, V. (2004) Communicating sad, bad, and difficult news in medicine, *Lancet,* 363: 312–19.

Fallowfield, L.J., Jenkins, V., Farewell, V., Saul, J., Duffy, A. and Eves, R. (2002) Efficacy of a Cancer Research UK communication skills training model for oncologists: a randomized controlled trial, *Lancet,* 359: 650–6.

Feinmann, J. (2002) Brushing up on doctors' communication skills, *Lancet,* 360: 1572.

Fellowes, D., Fallowfield, L.J., Saunders, C. and Houghton, J. (2001) Tolerability of hormone therapies for breast cancer: how informative are documented symptom profiles in medical notes for 'well tolerated' treatments? *Breast Cancer Research and Treatment,* 66: 73–81.

Feltham, C. (2005) Evidence-based psychotherapy and counselling in the UK: critique and alternatives, *Journal of Contemporary Psychotherapy,* 35(1): 131–43.

Finlay, I.G. and Watt, P. (1999) Randomized cross-over study of patient held records in oncology and palliative care, *Lancet,* 353: 558–9.

Fox, N.J. (2003) Practice-based evidence: towards collaborative and transgressive research, *Sociology,* 37(1): 81–102.

Friedrichsen, M.J., Strang, P.J. and Carlsson, M.E. (2002) Cancer patients' interpretations of verbal expressions when given information about ending cancer treatment, *Palliative Medicine,* 16: 323–30.

Gafni, A., Charles, C. and Whelan, T. (1998) The physician–patient encounter: the physician as a perfect agent for the patient versus the informed treatment decision-making model, *Social Science and Medicine,* 47: 347–54.

Garratini, S. and Garratini, L. (1993) Pharmaceutical prescribing in four European countries, *Lancet,* 342: 1191–2.

Gherardi, S. and Turner, B. (2002) Real men don't collect soft data, in A.M. Huberman and M.B. Miles (eds) *The Qualitative Researcher's Companion.* London: Sage.

Girgis, A., Sanson-Fisher, R.W. and Schofield, M.J. (1999) Is there consensus between breast cancer patients and providers on guidelines for breaking bad news? *Behavioural Medicine*, 25: 69–77.

Greenhalgh, T. (1999) Narrative based medicine in an evidence-based world, *British Medical Journal*, 318: 323–5.

Gunn, J., Southern, D., Chondros, P., Thomson, P. and Robertson, K. (2003) Guidelines for assessing postnatal problems: introducing evidence-based guidelines in Australian general practice, *Family Practice*, 20(4): 382–9.

Health Service Ombudsman for England (2003) *HSC Annual Report 2002–3*. Available at: http://www.health.ombudsman.org.uk/hsc/document/har03/har03.pdf (accessed 25 Dec. 2005).

Helseth, S. (2002) Help in times of crying: nurses' approach to parents with colicky infants, *Journal of Advanced Nursing*, 40(3): 267–74.

Holmberg, L., Baum, M. and Adami, H.O. (1999) On the scientific inference from clinical trials, *Journal of Evaluation in Clinical Practice*, 5(2): 157–62.

Jordan, B. and Jordan, C. (2000) *Social Work and the Third Way: Tough Love as Social Policy*. London: Sage.

Kim, M.K. and Alvi, A. (1999) Breaking the bad news of cancer: the patient's perspective, *Laryngoscope*, 109: 1064–7.

Kmietowicz, Z. (2005) Medical journals are corrupted by dependence on drug companies, *British Medical Journal*, 330: 1169.

Larner, G. (2004) Family therapy and the politics of evidence, *Journal of Family Therapy*, 26: 17–39.

Leo, J. and Cohen, D. (2003) Broken brains or flawed studies? A critical review of ADHD neuroimaging research, *Journal of Mind and Behavior*, 24(1): 29–56.

Levinson, W. and Roter, D.L. (1993) The effects of two continuing medical education programs on communication skills of practicing primary care physicians, *Journal of General Internal Medicine*, 8: 318–24.

Lovell, A., Zander, L. and James, C. (1987) The St Thomas's Hospital maternity case notes study: a randomized controlled trial to assess the effects of giving expectant mothers their own maternity case notes, *Paediatric and Perinatal Epidemiology*, 1: 57–66.

Macfarlane, A. (1992) Personal child health records held by parents, *Archives of Diseases of Childhood*, 67: 571–2.

Marwick, C. (2005) Complementary medicine must prove its worth, *British Medical Journal*, 330: 166.

Mauss, M. (1990) *The Gift: Forms and Functions of Exchange in Archaic Societies*. London: Routledge.

Miles, A., Grey, J.E., Polychronis, A. and Melchiorri, C. (2002) Critical advances in the evaluation and development of clinical care, *Journal of Evaluation in Clinical Practice*, 8: 87–102.

Mizrahi, T. (1984) Coping with patients, *Social Problems*, 32: 156–65.

National Audit Office (2005) *A Safer Place for Patients: Learning to Improve Patient Safety*. London: Stationery Office.

Oakley, A. (2000) *Experiments in Knowing: Gender and Method in the Social Sciences*. London: Polity Press.

Ollman, B. (2003) *Dance of the Dialectic: Steps in Marx's Method*. Chicago: University of Illinois Press.

Paul, F., Hendry, C. and Carrell, I.L. (2004) Meeting patient and relatives' information needs upon transfer from an intensive care unit: the development and evaluation of an information booklet, *Journal of Clinical Nursing*, 13: 396–405.

Payne, S., Kerr, C., Hawker, S., Hardey, M. and Powell, J. (2002) The communication of information about older people between health and social care practitioners, *Age and Ageing*, 31: 107–17.

Polanyi, M. (1983) *The Tacit Dimension*. Gloucester: Peter Smith.

Priest, H., Sawyer, A., Roberts, P. and Rhodes, S. (2005) A survey of interprofessional education in communication skills in health care programmes in the UK, *Journal of Interprofessional Care*, 19(3): 236–50.

Quirt, C.F., Mackillop, W.J. and Ginsburg, A.D. (1997) Do doctors know when their patients don't? A survey of doctor–patient communication in lung cancer, *Lung Cancer*, 18: 1–20.

Ramirez, A.J., Graham, J., Richards, M.A., Cull, A. and Gregory, W.M. (1995) Mental health of hospital consultants: the effects of stress and satisfaction of work, *Lancet*, 16: 724–8.

Rich, J.A. and Grey, C.M. (2003) Qualitative research on trauma surgery: getting beyond the numbers, *World Journal of Surgery*, 27: 957–61.

Roter, D.L., Hall, J.A. and Kern, D.E. (1995) Improving physicians' advance directives, patient and physician opinions regarding interviewing skills and reducing patients' emotional distress, *Archives of Internal Medicine*, 155: 1877–84.

Roter, D., Larson, S., Shinitsky, H. et al. (2004) Use of an innovative video feedback technique to enhance communication skills training, *Medical Education*, 38: 145–57.

Rowe, R., Garcia, J., McFarlane, A.J. and Davidson, L.L. (2001) Does poor communication contribute to stillbirths and infant deaths? A review, *Journal of Public Health Medicine*, 23(1): 23–34.

Rowe, R., Garcia, J., McFarlane, A.J. and Davidson, L.L. (2002) Improving communication between health professionals and women in maternity care: a structured review, *Health Expectations*, 5: 63–83.

Sackett, D.L., Rosenberg, W.M.C., Muir Grey, J.A., Haynes, R.B. and Richardson, W.S. (1996) Evidence-based medicine: what it is and what it isn't: it's about integrating individual clinical expertise and best external evidence, *British Medical Journal*, 312: 71–2.

Salmon, P. and Marchant-Haycox, S. (2000) Surgery in the absence of pathology: the relationship of patients' presentation to gynecologists' decisions for hysterectomy, *Journal of Psychosomatic Research*, 49: 119–24.

Sarangi, S. (2004) Towards a communicative mentality in medical and health care practice, *Communication and Medicine*, 1(1): 1–11.

Schön, D.A. (1991) *The Reflective Practitioner: How Professionals Think in Action*. London: Avebury.

Shaw, C., Williams, K.S. and Assassa, R.P. (2000) Patients' views of a new nurse-led continence service, *Journal of Clinical Nursing*, 9: 574–84.

Skelton, J.R. (2005) Everything you were afraid to ask about communication skills, *British Journal of General Practice*, 55(510): 40–6.

Skelton, J.R. and Hobbs, F.D.R. (1999) Descriptive study of cooperative language in primary care consultations by male and female doctors, *British Medical Journal*, 318: 576–9.

Smith, G.D., Hart, C., Blane, D., Gillis, C. and Hawthorne, V. (1997) Lifetime socio-economic position and mortality: prospective observational study, *British Medical Journal*, 314: 547.

Smith, R.C., Lyles, J.S., Mettler, J., Stoffelmayr, B.E. and Van Egeren, L.F. (1998) The effectiveness of intensive training for residents in interviewing: a randomized, controlled study, *Annals of Internal Medicine*, 128: 118–26.

Smith, S.D.M., Nicol, K.M., Devereux, J., Cornbleet, M.A. (1999) Encounters with doctors: quantity and quality? *Palliative Medicine*, 13: 217–23.

Stern, D.T., Linzer, M., O'Sullivan, P.S. and Weld, L. (1995) Evaluating medical students' literature-appraisal skills, *Academic Medicine*, 70: 152–4.

Sweeney, K.G. and Kernick. D. (2002) Clinical evaluation: constructing a new model for post-normal medicine, *Journal of Evaluation in Clinical Practice*, 8(2): 131–8.

Walter, F., Emery, J.D., Rogers, M. and Britten, M. (2004) Women's views of optimal risk communication and decision making in general practice consultations about the menopause and hormone replacement therapy, *Patient Education and Counselling*, 53(2): 121–8.

Whitstock, M.T. (2003) Seeking evidence from medical research consumers as part of the medical research process could improve the uptake of research evidence, *Journal of Evaluation in Clinical Practice*, 9(2): 213–24.

Widder, J. (2004) The origins of medical evidence: communication and experimentation, *Medicine, Health Care and Philosophy*, 7: 99–104.

3   Communicating effectively: what works for whom

Communicating 'effectively' for whom?

How can we define the success or failure of a communicative encounter? Is it concerned with whether it meets the goals of the people interacting? Is an encounter successful when a client's health outcomes are improved? Or is it an encounter that meets with broader organizational or institutional approval?

Whatever the answers to these questions, it is clear from a variety of authors that the achievement of 'good' communication is critical (Wensing et al. 1998). Not surprisingly, then, there has been considerable interest in the specific detail of the interactions between doctors and their patents and the potential effects that interaction style may have on patient outcomes (Kurtz et al. 1998). This interest has extended out from a medical focus to a whole range of health care domains and disciplines (Crawford et al 1998; Sarangi 2004).

The question of effective communication is central to any debate about health care and how a diverse client population may gain access to services. The construction of meaning is a complex process that moves beyond the simple roles of sender and receiver, as we have argued elsewhere (Crawford et al. 1998). Rather than merely encoding and decoding information (Osgood 1957) meaning may better be seen as the 'continuous interplay of perception and action in a co-regulated social context' (Fogel 1993: 15). Kagan (1998: 817) refers to the 'equation' of communication, where a delicate balance is maintained between the skills, experiences and resources that the interactants have available to draw upon. An imbalance occurs when one person experiences particular problems. These may be relatively 'mechanical' problems such as in the production or reception of speech, or with verbal comprehension, difficulties in formulating utterances or speech sounds or in using their available skills in different contexts with the range of other people encountered in health care (Law et al. 2005).

This chapter does not aim to offer specific advice about the conduct of clinical encounters. We will certainly see a fair amount of what others have recommended, but there are, as we shall see, many other sources which are more didactic in tone and the reader in search of advice might be better advised to consult these other volumes and articles. On the other hand, we will try to do something a little more challenging here. We shall invite the reader to think more critically about the issue of evidence-based communication and the issue of what is meant by effective communication. We will encourage consideration of the context of the communication, the kinds of culture and knowledge brought by the participants to the communicative encounter, the expectations, ideas and images which give it shape, form and meaning even before it has begun. We will also be interested in questions about whose interests are best served by 'effective communication'. What might be effective for clinicians is not necessarily effective for clients in the same way. They may have other agendas, plans and pleasures which are not necessarily well captured by the assumptions made in much health care communication research.

In connection with this we also aim to offer some suggestions as to how these questions of culture and context may best be understood theoretically, making contact once again with some of the issues we raised in Chapter 1 about the work of Foucault, Bourdieu, Beck and Giddens. The drift towards client-centred approaches in health care might be emancipatory and might allow the much maligned 'one size fits all' ethos in health care to be transcended, but on the other hand it retains a role for practitioners in stage managing the health care encounter, and makes the client or patient responsible for new things and new dimensions of the experience to which they are called upon to contribute.

The bigger picture: context, capital and troubling questions

Once we begin to follow this expanded picture so as to include disparities in knowledge and cultural resources that may exist between the interactants, communication difficulties become almost inevitable. One way of making sense of the disparities and differences between clients and practitioners in health care is through the issue of 'social capital'. As we mentioned in Chapter 1, issues concerned with differential access to knowledge, culture, language and resources can be captured with the notion of 'social capital'. Social capital consists of the stock of active connections among people: the trust, mutual understanding, and shared values and behaviours that bind the members of human networks and communities and make cooperative action possible (Cohen and Prusak 2001: 4).

In the conventional formulation of communication difficulties and the impediments they present to effective interaction in health care, it is believed that barriers arise from the 'mismatch between individual capacity for communication and the unmodified demands of the communication environment, leading to an increased risk of communication breakdown where service users' questions remain unanswered and diagnoses are insecure' (Law et al. 2005: 173). However, once we see this in terms of shared social capital a more socially embedded account of communication and its difficulties is possible. It is not just 'barriers' but the way the social world of the health care practitioner and the client are constructed. Often, it is assumed that the practitioner is rich in social capital, knowledge, training, equipment and the know-how to operate it; they may have legally mandated authority and greater social prestige. The client by contrast is often seen as lacking in social capital, knowledge, resources expertise and so on. Moreover, the recent interest in the socio-emotional aspects of care sees the client as lacking here too – as being somehow tremulous, anxious, apt to suffer depression, and needing a consulting room well-stocked with tissues. The idea of 'emotional capital' is relevant here. This was originated by Helga Nowotny who defined it as 'knowledge, contacts and relations as well as the emotionally valued skills and assets, which hold within any social network characterized at least partly by affective ties' (1981: 148). In advising practitioners to have tissues handy, as Boyle et al. (2004) do, we can see the implicit model of the client is being carefully constructed as someone who is apt to need them.

Clearly, clients and patients have many needs which health care providers should strive to address in an ideal world. We would certainly support the many attempts that are ongoing to increase the sensitivity of health care providers to this issue. However, it is equally important to tease out the assumptions which are made in some of these efforts and consider other ways in which communication may be constructed. If, for example, we see clients as being rich in cultural and emotional capital – for after all, they are often full of theories of their own about how their illnesses might work, and are continually devising coping strategies – we might well devise different ways of empowering them.

The approach we are suggesting also allows us to take a more critical line concerning what communication is about, or should be about in health care settings. For example, what should we expect the goals of the health care encounter to be? How do we know we've communicated effectively? In much conventional literature this question is taken for granted. There are many assertions as to the value of good or effective communication but the more politically nuanced question of whose interests will prevail in that communication is less well researched.

For example, it is common to read that 'effective communication between nurses and cancer patients is a central aspect of nursing care' (Wilkinson et al. 1998). Or that the psychosocial skills of health professionals exert a strong influence not only on patient satisfaction but also on compliance with medical advice and prescription plans. Moreover, more optimistic commentators such as Wilkinson et al. (1998) say it can also have a positive influence on health outcomes.

Note the kinds of phenomena that are foregrounded and privileged in these arguments. The positive, desirable outcomes are seen in terms of 'satisfaction' on the part of clients, whether they comply with advice and medication regimes, or whether they achieve a 'positive outcome'. Naturally, we are keen to see happy patients getting well. But here the terminology and outcome measures contain tacit theories about what is desirable. It is as if the outcome of 'effective communication' is patients who take their tablets as directed, indicate high levels of satisfaction on tick-box outcome measures and achieve a benign adjustment to their illness that is not overly troubling to health care providers or their families. The anodyne notion of 'satisfaction' sits oddly with the existentially critical issues which patients are sometimes facing. In what sense can a patient dying of cancer or AIDS be said to exhibit 'satisfaction'? Yet questionnaires measuring people's satisfaction are regularly administered to people in such situations as part of research and quality control procedures. It is hard not to wonder whether something crucial is being missed about the human condition and the state of health care.

Also, it is clear that patients themselves may sometimes have very different agendas as regards 'satisfaction' or 'compliance'. To illustrate this, let us relate a short anecdotal example. Some years ago one of us (BB) was doing fieldwork in a rural community in North Wales. Whereas the focus of the work was not related to medication compliance, it was intriguing that once rapport had been established, it became clear that among some groups of people prescription medication was a kind of currency. Of course, for many years it has been a matter of concern that people on drug treatment programmes have been selling their methadone, but these informants were using antidepressants and anti-anxiety drugs to exchange for babysitting services and tins of peas. The village was served by a mobile video library that came around once a week and videos could be obtained for tablets. Whereas common titles could be rented conventionally, if the proprietor was offered Kemadrine (procyclidine hydrochloride, a drug used to reduce the side effects of anti-schizophrenic medication) he provided pornographic videos from their hiding place under the front passenger seat in exchange.

Thus, from occasional vignettes into the role that prescription drugs and health care play in the life of communities it is possible to throw new light on the apparently straightforward matters of 'compliance' and 'satisfaction'. Compliance in conventional terms was clearly unsatisfactory, but the drugs were contributing to broader processes of sociality and network enhancement. Indeed, it is difficult to weigh up the costs and benefits exactly. We know that befriending schemes may be as effective as antidepressants in alleviating depression (Harris et al. 1999), but what about a visit from the video man?

As well as the therapeutic agendas to which some people in this community subscribed, which were strikingly different to those which are enjoined in health promotion materials and textbooks, other notions were awry. 'Satisfaction' was not solely about being communicated with according to good practice guidelines, but was for example the sense of having obtained more than one's prescription dose of medication by means of a ruse such as telling 'the surgery' that one had accidentally lost one's original tablets by putting them through the washing machine in a trouser pocket.

The point for our present discussion then is that the agendas, desires and forms of social capital of clients and practitioners may be more divergent than they might appear in the consulting room. This is not to say that the consulting room drama is in any simple sense 'false' or 'an act'. However, we should bear in mind the capacity of human beings to respond flexibly to situational cues and exhibit a wide ranging and at times seemingly contradictory set of repertoires where health (or anything else) is concerned. It has often been to the disadvantage of health care researchers that they have assumed a kind of 'honest soul' theory of persons, as if the interactants in health care were characters in a TV adaptation of a Charles Dickens novel (Potter and Wetherell 1987). Furthermore, to the extent that a person does not present an internally consistent account this is taken to be irrational or even bad behaviour. On the other hand if one adopts a more flexible view of the people involved as culturally adroit actors in the piece, this means that variation in a person's presentation of beliefs, behaviour and views is almost inevitable. Here people are expected to take up different subject positions available to them contingently, depending on the particular circumstances and situations available to them.

Interrogating the notion of effective communication: towards a critical re-reading of the literature

At first glance, the case for 'good communication', 'effective communication' and enhancing communicative skills of practitioners seems hard to dispute. The spectacle of taciturn, rude or maladroit practitioners leaving in their wake a string of distressed patients who are unlikely to comply with treatment recommendations is not an attractive one. Practitioners themselves say they want to become better communicators in the face of having to deal with patients in life-threatening situations, breaking bad news, and general consultation skills (Maguire and Pitceathly 2002). The case is, on the face of it, compelling. Good communication may improve patient recovery prospects whereas so called 'poor' communication may be distressing for patients, carers and practitioners and could have tragic consequences. The presence of 'effective' communication between clients and practitioners is a critical factor in the patient's perceived quality of care.

These concerns are in many ways commendable and represent a trend in research, education and practice to which we have contributed ourselves (Crawford et al. 1998). Moreover, government commitment to improving the 'emotional experience' of patients has been signalled in its recent publication *Now I Feel Tall* (Department of Health 2005). However, after nearly two decades of intensive activity it is time to take stock of what is happening and wonder aloud why so much research and education can co-exist with a situation in the UK which is marked not by satisfaction but increasing crisis in health care (Wilson 2004; Adams 2005; Allardyce 2005; Bosanquet et al. 2005).

Perhaps the answer to this is that the issue of communication in the health care consultation, and the question of 'what works for whom' is rather too narrowly focused. These issues depend in turn on the institutional settings within which communication takes place. A few minutes' thought about the health and social care services in the UK highlights how many of these involve different agencies sited in differing buildings, often many miles apart and between personnel who may be relative strangers to one another. Moreover, there is rapid turnover of staff in many health care services and a pervasive sense of time and resource pressure. As Brindle (2005) notes, people may express satisfaction with their local services but may have lost confidence in the way the NHS is run. The larger context then provides some of the reasons for the sense of crisis.

In addition, it may be that in cases where the situation is not unfolding according to the desires of the patients, health care workers and policymakers this is because larger scale structural factors are at work preventing it doing so.

It is fair to say that the majority, if not all, health care practitioners have received some level of training or guidance on how to communicate with service users. Across training curricula, future health professionals will be exposed to foundational knowledge and skills for interpersonal interaction, often including an introduction to counselling approaches. In addition, health care trainings tend to occur across the domains of academe and real-life practice environments. As such, the training takes cognizance of and affords assessment in the performance of communication skills, either directly or indirectly. We might wonder therefore why communication in health care has been sharply criticized in recent years. Is the training in communication skills inadequate? Are practitioners merely paying lip service to what makes for good communication, discarding this care dimension after qualifying? Or do health care settings themselves, and the way they are constructed, devalue and dis-inherit service users of what they require: clear, consistent, respectful and humane communication? Are health practitioners prevented from communicating effectively by the structures and systems that direct health care delivery? If this is the case, then a focus on the inadequacies of communication skills teaching, or the individual failure of practitioners to communicate effectively, might shift to the failure of environments to support effective communication.

Despite the acquisition of skills in training programmes, it cannot be guaranteed that practitioners will be able to apply them. This is particularly true when the patient is deemed to have communication difficulties and therefore the consultation cannot be dealt with in the time allocated. As Hemsley et al. (2001) note, one might hope that most practitioners could apply their laboriously acquired generic communication skills to good effect even when the patient has a disability that means they cannot speak. However, for several nurses in Hemsley and colleague's study, the amount of time required to communicate with patients with communication difficulties was a major limitation, as reflected in the following extract:

> You really don't have the time to stand there and wait for them to spit out their words; not having pens and papers; their frustrations – if they get so frustrated that they just give up, they say 'don't worry', it's a lost chance at communication I suppose.
>
> (p. 832)

The difficulty experienced in these circumstances is regrettable, and in some circumstances devastating for patients, but from our point of view also it is important to look at how the organizational features conspire against everyone's good intentions and desire to communicate. Even the very term 'clients with communication difficulties' is freighted with assumptions about where the problem lies. Underpinning this term, which is widely used in the literature, is the assumption that the difficulties lie with the client. This tends to pervade a good deal of thinking about clients with disabilities more generally and can also be detected in thinking about cases where the client is from a different culture and different language community than the professional.

Now, as even a fleeting familiarity with the disability studies literature will remind us, the identification of where problems are in the system of disablement is controversial. If the problems are identified as being inside or belonging to the person experiencing them, this is often associated with a very medicalized and individualized approach to disability. This kind of thinking often involves seeing disability as a kind of personal tragedy that has randomly befallen the person.

Thus, when we read about 'communication impairment' and see the term applied to people with disabilities in clinical settings, it is as well to bear these arguments in mind, and ask ourselves the question of just who is being problematized here?

Institutional and organizational factors in communicative failure

No matter how we conceptualize the issue of disability, however, there are clearly problems which may preoccupy and sometimes overwhelm carers, clients and practitioners. The question is whether we see the person suffering the problems as being disabled or whether we see the institutional or societal context as causing the problems to be exposed. The relevance of this to the issue of effective communication is that the question goes well beyond the skills, intentions, and affective and cognitive organization of the practitioners and patients, but is embedded in the cultural resources which we have to draw upon and the institutions within which suffering and healing are framed and within which they are undertaken. The sense that the problems lie within the patient, or that patients who are, outside the clinic, active and resourceful in their coping strategies are somehow deficient or vulnerable are both borne from the culture or context of health care as much as from the people within it.

This focus on institutional contexts and the institutional ethos is highlighted by studies of disability, but it becomes more contentious still when we consider the issues of race and ethnicity. Here the question of institutionally embedded prejudices and assumptions made by service planners and policymakers becomes especially crucial. This may well happen despite attempts at an interpersonal level to empower the consumer. Because of broader patterns of inequality in society as a whole there may be limitations on the extent to which consumers can empower themselves. As Rutherford et al. (2005) highlight, there have been a number of policy-based and managerial changes in the health service which have supposedly been designed to change the emphasis of the way it is managed. A consistent theme in the manifest position of policymakers is that greater authority and decision-making power should be permitted to patients and frontline staff, as described for example in the Department of Health publication *Shifting the Balance of Power* (2000). Another example is the document *Developing Key Roles for Nurses and Midwives* (Department of Health 2003), which describes how nurses and midwives will play a key role in achieving a patient-centred future. Indeed, in many policymaking circles there have been attempts to move away from what has been called 'one size fits all' health and social care (Boon et al. 2004). There is a growing emphasis on tailoring service approaches to client needs.

However, race, ethnicity and racism present a notable suite of issues where the proverbial playing field could not easily be described as level and the question of 'effective communication' is a problematic one. To illustrate this, let us consider the much-publicized case of David 'Rocky' Bennett, a black man who died tragically while being restrained by nurses at the Norvic Clinic in Norfolk, England in October 1998. The Inquiry report (Blofeld et al. 2003) conceded that he had been 'treated kindly' during his stays in hospital, but at the same time notes that there had been several occasions when he was subject to racial taunts and abuse which were not dealt with appropriately at the time. From the point of view of our concern with communication, however, the most crucial issues come from its treatment of racial inequality in the UK's National Health Service. Describing the organization as a whole as 'institutionally racist' (p. 41), Blofeld and colleagues go on:

> Many witnesses told us that the black and minority ethnic community have a very real fear of the Mental Health Service. They fear that if they engage with the mental health services they will be locked up for a long time, if not for life, and treated with medication which may eventually kill them.
>
> (p. 42)

Thus as the report goes on to note, there have been difficulties in establishing communication between health care practitioners and organizations and members of the communities in question. This issue has been subject to scrutiny from other bodies too. In a census of the position of different ethnic groups in the UK's health service (Kennedy and Patel 2005), it emerged that black people are three times more likely than average to be admitted to a hospital for mentally ill people, and they are 44 per cent more likely to be detained under the Mental Health Act. Black Caribbean patients are twice as likely to be referred through the courts; black African patients almost twice as likely to be referred to mental health services through the police; black and Indian patients 50 per cent more likely to be placed in seclusion once in hospital; and black Caribbean men 29 per cent more likely to experience incidents involving physical restraint.

Now the relevance of all this for the subject of communication and the question of how to communicate effectively is to do with the crucial question of context. Under circumstances like these it is very difficult for participants in any given health encounter to create a mutually empowering space for interaction, no matter how well motivated to do so. If an institution tends to act more coercively towards one section of the population than others then this affects the nature of the communication that can take place. This is a theme to which we shall return in later chapters, but for the time being it should suffice to alert the reader to the situational and contextual constraints on communication in health care settings and to consider just in whose interests communication is likely to be effective. Later, we shall also be examining some specific strategies to change this.

Breaking new ground: cybermedicine and the communicative encounter

There are a variety of new factors that give shape and form to the communication which is possible in health care encounters. As well as changes in the attitudes, lifestyles, family structures and patterns of work and unemployment an increasing proportion of people are living at least part of their life through electronic media. The time when diagnoses, treatments and even operations being conducted over computerized links which more enthusiastic proponents were predicting in the mid-1990s is still some distance away. However, information, advice and potential for interaction with like-minded colleagues, fellow sufferers and 'cyberfriends' has grown dramatically since the mid-1990s.

Health care practitioners have often found themselves competing with other sources of information which are perceived as more credible and leave a more lasting impression. In a recent study Nielsen et al. (2005) found that other than health professionals, alternative sources of information most used are friends, relatives and the Internet. Interpersonal influences and communications have been identified as crucial factors by many scholars of the diffusion of innovations and new ideas (Rogers 2003). What is more interesting from the point of view of scholars of health in the twenty-first century is the way the role of the Internet has increased, which has been identified by many authors (Jejurikar et al. 2002). From the point of view of medical practitioners looking at this information though, the standards of accuracy and relevance are believed to be poor. From the practitioner's point of view they may, as Nielsen et al. (2005) describe, try to seek out and 'correct' the 'misconceptions' as part of the consultation. However, the development of Internet health, or as Nettleton and Burrows (2003) have called it 'e-scaped medicine', has a substantial and increasing influence on clients, and how they conceptualize their distress and attempt to act upon it via encounters with flesh and blood health professionals.

One of the most significant phenomena to emerge with the burgeoning of electronically mediated health is the growth in opportunities for interaction and electronic or virtual communities, noted increasingly from the mid-1990s onwards (Wellman 1997). Indeed it may be that these virtual communities can be seen as important sources of 'self-help' support, facilitated through electronic media. Eyesenbach et al. (2004) note that it is remarkably difficult to show evidence of a positive effect of this kind of communication. People often accessed these facilities in conjunction with other sorts of therapy or support, so it is hard to tell whether any improvement was due solely to the Internet support. Sometimes an association between greater use of peer-to-peer groups and better outcomes can be observed, but we are still unclear whether increased use leads to better outcomes, or whether an improved prognosis due to other factors leads to increased use.

Malone et al. (2004) sought to discern the impact of this on health professionals and their consultations with clients. Whereas their survey disclosed that 75 per cent of the health professionals questioned had been consulted by a patient bearing information obtained from the Internet, only a minority (5 per cent) had experienced this more than six times a month. However, there were some powerful mixed feelings about patients bringing such information to the encounter. In many cases, especially when patients had hazarded a diagnosis of their own and investigated possible courses of treatment, this was seen as a bad thing. Health professionals often had to admit their relative ignorance to Internet-informed patients and offered them follow-up consultations later; yet this was unsatisfactory because it meant more work. Admitting ignorance in the consultation itself amounted to a professional 'loss of face' and a feeling of being 'disempowered' or even 'professionally insecure' (p. 191). Childs (2004) on the other hand reports a somewhat more favourable picture, where some survey evidence can be found which suggests that the majority of patients and about half of professionals found it helpful to discuss material on the Internet. This then offers a new potential for health care providers to be co-explorers of the electronic landscape with the client.

Words of advice: the implications of communication study for health care encounters

A great many educators, practitioners and researchers have sought to address the question of how best we might advise the rising generation of health care practitioners who will spend their lives communicating with clients. This has ranged between slim volumes of avuncular advice to intensive training programmes with video feedback and assessed role-playing exercises, to a present-day fascination with virtual patients in computer-simulated consulting rooms so as to measure variables such as the amount of eye contact made.

In a volume which is by now a classic, *The Doctor's Communication Handbook*, Peter Tate (2001) counsels readers to be attentive to patients, with an emphasis on listening to and observing the patient, and advises practitioners to delay hypothesizing or drawing conclusions too early. Tate also emphasizes trying to view illness from the patient's perspective. Whereas these kinds of edicts sound relatively straightforward, putting them meaningfully into practice may be rather difficult: 'Every patient is unique, and that is why medicine is so difficult to teach and to learn'. While there is an exhortation for practitioners to share understanding of problems with patients, this is seen to have limitations: 'Doctors are good at giving explanations ... the fly in the ointment is that patients are bad at understanding them'. When doctors provide information they frequently do so in an inflexible way governed by their own agenda rather than what individual patients wish to know. According to Silverman et al. (1998) they tend not to check whether patients have understood what they have been told.

Preparing the ground

Boyle et al. (2004) note that for patients entering specialist clinics and units after having been seen by their family physician, a good many of their expectations and orientations have already been set up. Referring doctors and office staff can profoundly influence the experience of treatment by means of the orientation they give to the patient and help patients understand the world they are entering. Effective early orientation, according to Boyle and colleagues, includes issues such as appropriate expectations. Patients and referring doctors may wish to explore the expertise of secondary services to which they are entrusting their wellbeing, so information about skills, areas of specialization and the facilities available might be desirable. First impressions are believed to be important (Henman et al. 2002). This begins with reception staff, who act as gatekeepers to the practice or clinic and set the tone. The setup of the consulting rooms needs to allow shared information, for example diagrams, reports and other aids to be readily visible to the patient. In the event of the news being bad, having chairs close enough together to comfort a distressed patient might be desirable. These concerns on the part of Boyle et al. (2004) about the physical aspects of the facilities are particularly apposite in relation to ongoing concern in the UK about the cleanliness of hospitals. A recent audit by the Healthcare Commission (2005) based on a study of 99 UK hospitals found that only one-third met appropriately high standards of cleanliness, whereas others showed evidence of room for improvement and 22, many of which were mental health care facilities, had 'serious widespread problems in relation to cleanliness'. These kinds of problems affect the level of confidence patients and their carers have in the service they are receiving. As well as the physical condition of the clinical setting the emotional climate can give some important cues to the incoming patients and relatives. Boyle et al. (2004) recommend staff who smile, welcome patients, explain delays and assist patients in solving problems. This might sound trite, yet the climate of a successful health care encounter can be set by the initial welcome given to patients as they arrive. Patients can be traumatized by seeing their surgeon's spontaneous reaction to a scan that shows progressive disease, for example. An acquaintance tells us of an incident when he inadvertently upset a patient by muttering, 'that's appalling' when he was in fact referring to the photographic quality of the X rays.

Eliciting patients' problems and concerns

Making a positive opening is recommended, with smiles and eye contact (Maguire and Pitceathly 2002), as well as welcoming patients by name (Boyle et al. 2004). Maintaining eye contact at reasonable intervals through the consultation helps to show interest (Goldberg et al. 1993). If the patient is already known to be suffering from an illness, for example if they have received a diagnosis of cancer, Boyle et al. (2004) recommend acknowledging the impact this will have had on the patient. One study (Fogarty et al. 1999) showed that 30 seconds at the beginning of the consultation spent highlighting that this was a difficult time and that the staff would be there to help the patient, significantly reduced patient anxiety. Encouraging patients to be exact about the sequence in which their problems occurred, the dates of key events and their perceptions and feelings is recommended by Maguire and Pitceathly (2002). This assists patients in remembering their experiences, feeling understood (Cox et al. 1981) and in coping with their problems.

A further strategy is to use what Boyle et al. (2004: 478) call 'creating gaps': 'If you don't make a big enough opening, important pathology may be missed'. As Maguire and Pitceathly (2002) advise, it is important to elicit patients' main concerns, yet up to 60 per cent of cancer patients' concerns remain undisclosed, even in hospice settings where slower turnover of staff and patients might facilitate relationships and make disclosure more likely.

Many cases of miscommunication leading to complaint occur when one or both parties are tired or distracted (Hickson et al. 1994). It is also recommended that practitioners ask patients what they understand the problem to be and what information they want so as to tailor consultations accordingly, and asking 'is there anything else?' before changing topic or ending the consultation.

Promoting interaction between patient and practitioner is believed to be desirable. Boyle et al. (2004) suggest indicating that questions are welcome and giving the patient time to process and respond. They also recommend letting patients tell their own story; as they will often have rehearsed it ahead of time and wish to divulge. At this stage in the consultation, it is recommended that interruptions from the practitioner are minimized, and that in the long term this will enhance satisfaction and efficiency. In one study, doctors on average re-directed the patient's opening statements within 23.1 seconds; thus the initial statement of concerns was only completed in 28 per cent of cases (Marvel et al. 1999). This tendency to try to 'fix' things by offering advice and reassurance is a common stratagem or 'routine' in health care, as Maguire and Pitceathly (2002) note. One study of New York general practitioners found that they interjected with advice and reassurance within 18 seconds of patients mentioning the first problem (Beckman and Frankel 1984) which means that patients are less apt to disclose difficulties in the future. These problems in eliciting patients' concerns and in tailoring information to their individual needs perhaps contribute to the high rate of affective disorders in patients with cancer. Despite its high prevalence, only half of those with depression are recognized and treated appropriately (Hardman et al. 1989).

Thus, the use of 'active listening' to clarify what patients are concerned about has been widely promoted in the literature (Maguire et al. 1996) – that is, clarifying and exploring any hints about problems and distress. At the same time, however, interruptions are discouraged, especially before patients have completed important statements. Borrowing from techniques used in client-centred counselling, summarizing and paraphrasing the patient's account shows patients they have been heard, and gives them the chance to clarify any misunderstandings (Maguire et al. 1996).

The display of empathy will show that the practitioner has a sense of how the patient might be feeling. Maguire and Pitceathly (2002) also recommend that practitioners feed back to patients their intuitions about what the patient may be feeling ('you say you are coping well, but I get the impression you are struggling with this treatment'). This is a technique of emotion work called 'templating' – laying out a culturally intelligible structure or 'template' for the patient. Even if the guess is incorrect, enthusiasts for this technique say that it shows patients that the practitioner is trying to further their understanding of the problem. Maguire and Pitceathly are particularly keen that doctors should not engage in what they call 'blocking' (p. 698). This may include offering advice and reassurance before the main problems have been identified, explaining away distress as normal, attending merely to physical aspects of the condition, switching the topic, especially when things get awkward, and 'jollying' patients along. Nielsen et al.'s (2005) work suggests that eliciting a patient's expectations about what they anticipate from the consultation and subsequent treatment as a routine part of the consultation could help to improve communication and satisfaction.

Critical conditions: unpacking the meaning of emotionally enhanced encounters

While all this advice about the structure of clinical encounters, the communicative strategies and the emotional tone adds to the repertoire of the practitioner, and enhances the range of emotional matters he or she can deal with, it is worth noting how this is also urging a change in the nature of medical communication. The practitioner is now responsible for ordering and domesticating the patient's psychoemotional landscape. Rather than being private matters for the patient and his or her loved ones, the emotional adjustments to illness are the territory of the physician, the nurse or the counsellor. These developments in the literature about health care communication, and the advice and training provided to practitioners are not merely about the skills of the practitioner. They are also in important senses about the kind of person the practitioner should be, the kind of patient they should have and the role of emotions in public and private. In a curious sense this movement in education and training for health care practitioners reflects a broader trend towards more floridly wrought and publicly expressed displays of emotion in civic life, as West (2004) identifies. Indeed, it could be suggested that these psychotherapeutic ambitions are, in a sense, cultivating vulnerability (Furedi 2004). Problems of culture, of one's impending death (often with great pain and loss of dignity) or with the inequalities which mean that some groups die sooner than others, can be repackaged in terms which are psychological rather than economic, theological, philosophical or cultural.

While there is clearly much to be welcomed in the spectacle of doctors caring for the wellbeing of their charges in a well-rounded manner, this 'orthopaedics of the soul' (Miller and Rose 1994) is expanding the territory of the health care professions into new areas. We are left wondering about the fate of the patient with cancer who would prefer to retain his or her experiences of the disease as private matters. Experiences of devastation, grief or rage may be considered inappropriate for a health care consultation which is unlikely to exceed ten minutes. Will they be exhorted ever more zealously to emote by communication with skills-trained practitioners? We are not contending that there is a single best way to deal with these things. Rather, the point is to ensure that the reader is aware of what is at stake. This is not just the technical matter of ensuring good communication, but is part of a more moral and political project which extends medicine into new territories of emotionality.

This involves suturing together the eminently sensible ideas and attaching to them a good many largely unexamined moral, political and existential implications. This kind of process can also be seen when we look at the issue of 'information'. This might seem a relatively innocent issue since few would dispute the need for information – it underlies the notion of informed consent for example. Yet even here we can see the operation of assumptions concerning the nature of the information available and the nature of patients and the way they learn. We are, for example, enjoined to ask patients what information they would like, and to prioritize their 'information needs' so that the more pressing needs can be satisfied first if time is short. We are encouraged to present information by category, for example by using approved forms of phrase, such as 'you said you would like to know the nature of your illness'. Informed by notions of good practice in the education system, practitioners are advised to make sure the patient has understood before they move on (Ley 1988). With complex illnesses or treatments, it might be desirable for practitioners to check if the patient would like additional information; here, some practitioners have experimented with written information sheets, audiotapes and various kinds of computer media. However, as Maguire and Pitceathly (2002) caution, if the patient has a poor prognosis, providing media of this kind might facilitate despair rather than positive coping. Even so, it is considered appropriate to properly inform patients of treatment options, and whether they want to be involved in decisions. Patients taking part in decision making are more likely to adhere to treatment plans (Silverman et al. 1998).

What we have said about the health care professional's incursions into the emotional aspects of care can equally well be said of the professional's control of the informational world of the client. As Contu et al. (2003) note sceptically, when we talk of 'information' or 'learning' we are very often mobilizing the terms in a way that legitimizes and reinforces a neo-liberal ethos, as an inescapable answer to the newly liberalized markets in health care and the changing times of the supposedly knowledge driven, globalized economy. In a broader sense, information is the handmaid of league tables, performance targets and globalized health tourism. What is most striking is how the discourses of 'learning' and 'information' seem to have become constituted as truth: it is assumed that information and learning, like vitamins and stopping smoking, are unproblematically *good things*. There is however a more critical line which could be taken and which has been widely explored in sociology and organization theory (Rose 1990; Contu et al. 2003). This involves understanding such humanistically informed management of patients and disease as part of a more subtle and disingenuous form of control. These apparently enlightened practices are entangled in making and enforcing notions of the person that require him or her to 'take responsibility' (Newnes and Radcliffe 2005) as part of neo-liberal and other hegemonic forms of health care, the organization of health care work, economy and subjectivity.

A further difficulty with these approaches is that the activities which are deemed desirable are often described as if they were part of a generic skill set that could be applied to almost any health care encounter. A good deal of the foregoing has been derived from studies of people with cancer and in trying to identify what works for whom, as we promised in the title of this chapter, we are sometimes left with more questions than answers. In striving to be useful, researchers have sometimes become so bland and generic as to say little more than the obvious. One way of making this point is to imagine what would happen if we inverted the advice and suggested instead that they should not make eye contact, should not greet patients with a smile, should interrupt them and not give them a chance to ask questions.

As Maguire and Pitceathly (2002) note, current evidence suggests that attending workshops or courses, combined with opportunities to receive feedback about their communication in real consultations, will allow practitioners to learn most. From the outset of the present concern with communication skills in health care it appeared that training programmes for doctors which were demonstrably effective, were usually of an eclectic style and integrated a communication skills curriculum into clinical practice over a period of time.

As a result of these activities, it is believed that both practitioners and patients will benefit. Patients will disclose more concerns, perceptions and feelings about their predicament, will feel less distressed, and be more satisfied. Practitioners on the other hand will feel more confident about how they are communicating and obtain more validation from patients. These benefits bear a curious resemblance to a sales pitch, inasmuch as the benefits seem to be targeted to the kinds of issues that practitioners are presumed to be concerned about, maximizing their information gain, boosting their satisfaction ratings and avoiding stress and burnout. In a sense then, they are imbued with triumphalism.

Constraints and confines: contextual difficulties in achieving effective communication

Despite the recommendations for effective communicative practice of the kind we have already seen, there are other aspects of the institutional context which militate against the achievement of these communicative ideals. One of the most pressing issues is that of time. In Law et al.'s (2005) study of communication between health care professionals and clients who had communication difficulties there were a number of concerns and considerations over the issue of time. An overwhelming awareness of time pressure in the consultation prompted some carers to suggest that the service user himself or herself was being used as a time-saving device at the expense of more meaningful clinical interaction. For example, some felt that time was wasted because the practitioner did not make full use of the patient's notes, putting unnecessary strain on the interaction by requesting redundant information:

> So they don't have time to discover each person's particular way of com-
> municating, which is bullshit ... the time they waste repeating themselves
> and asking questions could be spent in those first five minutes discovering
> something about that person and then supporting that conversation, and this
> is what these GPs and receptionists need to learn. (Carer/aphasia)
>
> (Law et al. 2005: 177)

Clearly, lack of time is a common concern in primary care. This, combined with the special difficulties faced by people with communication difficulties, may be especially important for this client group because the status of the interaction is particularly vulnerable.

In line with accepted practice in health care education, Maguire and Pitceathly (2002) are convinced of the value of role-playing exercises in correcting what they see to be the major problems. Practising communication skills with simulated patients helps develop communicative competence and leads to less so-called 'blocking behaviour'. Nevertheless there remain concerns that practitioners trained in this way might not transfer these learned skills to clinical practice as might be hoped. Maguire and Pitceathly suggest using 'real' consultations as vehicles for feedback and discussion of skills as this might enable more effective skill transfer.

Despite the effectiveness of skill transfer, it is important to bear in mind that the effectiveness of communication depends on contextual factors which will influence whether or not the health professional has anything to communicate. For example, in the UK, the GP, working in a primary care practice, is often the first point of contact for much health care for many people. Unless the pain or injury is catastrophic, in which case the person may go directly to hospital, the GP is not only the first point of contact but also mediates between the patient and secondary services. Whereas a patient with unexplained pains and lumps in the abdomen may be referred to secondary services for further investigations and treatment, often the main point of communication with the patient is still the GP. The liaison between GPs and their colleagues in the primary care practice and the secondary, specialist services has often been a source of concern.

To explore the workings of communication then, and examine how this may succeed or fail, we need to understand the communicative networks behind the consultation. A 'successful' meeting between a GP and a patient depends on a good deal of communication having gone on beforehand in order for the patient and his or her condition to be managed in a way which appears appropriate and sympathetic. To consider this question in more detail let us examine a study by Farquhar et al. (2005) of communication between professionals caring for women with ovarian cancer. Ovarian cancer is a relatively common ailment in women and tends to be progressive with low survival rates; five years after diagnosis only 30 per cent of sufferers are expected to be alive (Office for National Statistics 1999). The diffuse presenting symptoms mean that it often escapes diagnosis until the disease is well advanced. The speed at which the disease advances means that prompt investigation and treatment are believed to be desirable once the disease is suspected. Yet as Farquhar et al. (2005) describe, sometimes communication in this respect is far from fluent:

> ... we can end up losing track with them because if they are going over to [the hospital] once a week ... then they haven't really got the time or inclination often to come and see us as well. Well that's fair enough and I don't want to impose ... But it does make communication, an immediate communication rather than a letter coming through 3 weeks later, [important].
>
> (p. 362)

Getting information from hospital consultants through to GPs can be complicated. Even something as apparently simple as a letter from the hospital to the GP could be problematic and subject to delay. When the letters eventually come it may leave the GP little the wiser. As one of Farquhar and colleagues's participants was quoted as saying:

> If you get a hospital discharge when they are hand written they are often illegible or copies ... The copies can be very, very faint. They can sometimes have a list of results but no actual list of a plan, and what patients have been told ... What I really need to know is what the patient has been told and what the plan is, and possibly even a guarded prognosis ... because obviously that makes a big difference on how I can contribute.
>
> (p. 363)

Thus, even in the case of a problem which all parties agree is urgent and which involves two institutions – the GP's practice and the specialist oncology clinic – the pathways of communication can be problematic. Thus, if GPs are hesitant, or appear to be ill-informed about a patient's case this may well be disturbing for the patient, but is part and parcel of the way services work. The point of describing this example in detail is that it is emblematic of the problems that occur in communication between services and agencies, and it highlights the need to see the broader institutional context. A practitioner who is under-informed, frustrated by the paucity of communication or does not know how much the client has been told already may not be in a good position to make a positive impression, however well-developed their own individual communicative style might be.

In a study by Manias et al. (2005) of nurses acquiring a professional identity, while some participants indicated that they felt comfortable asking doctors why particular medications were prescribed for patients, a number of others said they did not actively seek medication information from doctors because they were not readily available and sometimes their knowledge did not appear to be as detailed and as wide ranging as had been expected. Indeed, participants commented that when they asked, they were told to look up the information in reference texts anyway.

Sometimes the aspects of communication in which practitioners might be concerned are outside the bounds of what researchers generally study in the West. For example, Stott (2004) describes how communication interventions in developing nations in Africa have utilized other kinds of media. Here, as he points out, a good deal of the most effective health care interventions are not necessarily ones which need a lot of complex scientific research. Indeed 'seeds and agricultural equipment are better for health than bandages' (p. 1193). Equally, the effectiveness of some of the more vital interventions is well known, but the trick is to disseminate them. Salt and sugar solutions have had a big effect on mortality from diarrhoea. Getting the message across is difficult. How do we reach thousands of poor people who may be widely distributed across large rural areas and whose understanding of their body and its functions may be at odds with western medicine? Stott describes interventions such as play acting, with motivated local people playing all the parts, as a powerful medium of communication tool. 'Africa can teach us that we need to pay proper regard to different approaches to communication' (p. 1193).

Conclusion: towards reflective effectiveness

In conclusion then, it is appropriate to reprise the key points of the chapter. We hope that we have encouraged the reader to consider a number of questions when thinking about the issue of whether communication is effective. Chief among these is the question of who benefits from 'effective' communication. After all, patients and practitioners may have different agendas.

A further consideration which we have attempted to introduce for the reader is the necessity of making sense of the increasing desire of practitioners and those who educate them to expand their sphere of influence and expertise into the client's emotional life. Now there is not necessarily a right or wrong answer to this question – after all, it is debatable as to what exactly is fair game for the therapeutic intervention – but it is a movement which we should at least contemplate to ensure that we are comfortable with its implications.

The communicative skills of the effective practitioner are simply stated. Indeed, at core they often seem to be little more than the common courtesies we would extend to a friend or work colleague. Greeting people, giving them our attention, looking up from our notes or computer screen at them while they are talking to us, being courteous and allowing them to feel that they've been listened to may seem self-evident, even banal. The challenge then is not merely to define them, but to ensure that they are inculcated in a way which is robust in the face of organizational and institutional pressures which predispose rudeness and perfunctory treatment. The biomedical interventions available may be much the same, and sometimes, sadly we can offer little hope to clients. Yet there is a world of difference between clients who feel they have been cared for and looked after and those who do not. Beyond the consulting room, this extends outward to broader questions of trust and confidence of the public in the health professions and to whether public opinion is supportive of the institutions and professions designed to provide health care services.

Finally, it is important to note that there may be situational, geographical and organizational constraints on the communications which can take place. No matter how acutely developed the consultation skills are, the results may not come back from the laboratory in time, the information from colleagues may not have been forth-coming and the time available to establish rapport with the client may be minimal. These kinds of constraints mean that the practitioner must be a very versatile com-municator indeed. Notions of competent, effective communication as they stand at the moment may be very crude instruments indeed to capture the mix of flexibility and compassion that may be necessary in such circumstances.

References

Adams, C. (2005) NHS cash crisis 'eroding confidence', *Financial Times*, 8 December.

Allardyce, J. (2005) NHS 24 helpline putting patients' health at risk, *Sunday Times*, 3 April.

Beckman, A.B. and Frankel, R.M. (1984) The effect of physician behaviour on the collection of data, *Annals of Internal Medicine,* 101: 692–6.

Blofeld, J., Sallah, D., Sashidharan, S., Stone, R. and Struthers, J. (2003) *David Bennett: An Independent Inquiry Set up under HSG (24) 97*. London: Department of Health.

Boon, H., Verhoef, M., O'Hara, D. and Findlay, B. (2004) From parallel practice to inte-grative health care: a conceptual framework, *Bio Med Central Health Services Research*. Available at http://www.biomedcentral.com/1472–6963/4/15 (accessed 20 December 2005).

Bosanquet, N., De Zoete, H. and Beuhler, E. (2005) *The NHS in 2010: Reform or Bust*. London: Reform Research Trust.

Boyle, F.M., Robinson, E., Heinrich, P. and Dunn, S.M. (2004) Cancer: communicating the team game, *Australia and New Zealand Journal of Surgery*, 74: 477–81.

Brindle, D. (2005) Society: view from the top – rating customer satisfaction is no easy task, *Guardian*, 7 September.

Childs, S. (2004) Surveys of usage of the health Internet: part one, *Health Information on the Internet*, 39: 1.

Cohen, D. and Prusak, L. (2001) *In Good Company: How Social Capital Makes Organizations Work*. Boston, MA.: Harvard Business School Press.

Contu, A., Grey, C. and Ortenblad, A. (2003) Against learning, *Human Relations*, 56(8): 931–52.

Cox, A., Hopkinson, K. and Rutter, N. (1981) Psychiatric interviewing techniques. II. Nat-uralistic study: eliciting factual information, *British Journal of Psychology*, 138: 283–91.

Crawford, P., Brown, B. and Nolan, P. (1998) *Communicating Care: Language in Health Care Contexts*. Cheltenham: Stanley Thornes.

Department of Health (DoH) (2000) *Shifting the Balance of Power*. London: Stationery Office.

Department of Health (DoH) (2003) *Developing Key Roles for Nurses and Midwives: A Guide for Managers*. London: Stationery Office.

Department of Health (DoH) (2005) *Now I Feel Tall: What a Patient-led NHS Feels Like*. London: Department of Health.

Eyesenbach, G., Powell, J., Englesakis, M., Rizo, C. and Stern, A. (2004) Health related virtual communities and electronic support groups: systematic review of the effects of online peer to peer interactions, *British Medical Journal*, 328: 1166–72.

Farquhar, M.C., Barclay, S.I.G., Earl, H., Grande, G.F., Emery, J. and Crawford, R.A.F. (2005) Barriers to effective communication across the primary/secondary interface: examples from the ovarian cancer patient journey (a qualitative study), *European Journal of Cancer Care*, 14: 359–66.

Fogarty, L.A., Curbow, B.A., Wingard, J.R., McDonnell, K. and Somerfield, M.R. (1999) Can 40 seconds of compassion reduce patient anxiety? *Journal of Clinical Oncology*, 17: 371–9.

Fogel, A. (1993) Two principles of communication: co-regulation and framing, in J. Nadel and L. Camaioni (eds) *New Perspectives in Communication Development*. London: Routledge.

Furedi, F. (2004) *Therapy Culture: Cultivating Vulnerability in an Uncertain Age*. London: Routledge.

Goldberg, D.P., Jenkins, L., Miller, T. and Farrier, E.B. (1993) The ability of trainee general practitioners to identify psychological distress among their patients, *Psychological Medicine*, 23: 185–93.

Hardman, A., Maguire, P. and Crowther, D. (1989) The recognition of psychiatric morbidity on a medical oncology ward, *Journal of Psychosomatic Research*, 33: 235–9.

Harris, T., Brown, G.W. and Robinson, R. (1999) Befriending as an intervention for chronic depression among women in an inner city, *British Journal of Psychiatry*, 174: 219–24.

Healthcare Commission (2005) *A Report on Hospital Cleanliness in England*. London: Commission for Health Care Audit and Inspection.

Hemsley, B., Sigafoos, J., Balandin, S. et al. (2001) Nursing the patient with severe communication impairment, *Journal of Advanced Nursing*, 35(6): 827–35.

Henman, M.J., Butow, P.N., Brown, R.F., Boyle, F. and Tattersall, M.H. (2002) Lay constructions of decision-making in cancer, *Psycho-oncology*, 11: 295–306.

Hickson, G.B., Clayton, E.W. and Entman, S.S. (1994) Obstetricians' prior malpractice experience and patients' satisfaction with care, *Journal of the American Medical Association*, 272: 1583–7.

Jejurikar, S.S., Rovak, J.M., Kuzon, W.M., Chung, K.C., Kotsis, S.V. and Cederna, P.S. (2002) Evaluation of plastic surgery information on the Internet, *Annals of Plastic Surgery*, 49: 460–5.

Kagan, A. (1998) Supported conversation for adults with aphasia: methods and resources for training conversation partners, *Aphasiogy*, 12: 817–30.

Kennedy, I. and Patel, K. (2005) *Count Me In: Results of a National Census of Inpatients in Mental Health Hospitals and Facilities in England and Wales*. London: Commission for Health Care Audit and Inspection.

Kurtz, S., Silverman, J. and Draper, J. (1998) *Teaching and Learning Communication Skills in Medicine*. Oxford: Radcliffe Medical Press.

Law, J., Bunning, J., Byng, S., Farrelly, S. and Heyman, B. (2005) Making sense in primary care: leveling the playing field for people with communication difficulties, *Disability and Society*, 20(2): 169–84.

Ley, P. (1988) *Communication with Patients: Improving Satisfaction and Compliance*. London: Croom Helm.

Maguire, P. and Pitceathly, F. (2002) Key communication skills and how to acquire them, *British Medical Journal*, 325: 697–700.

Maguire, P., Faulkner, A., Booth, K., Elliott, C. and Hillier, V. (1996) Helping cancer patients to disclose their concerns, *European Journal of Cancer*, 32a: 78–81.

Malone, M., Harris, R., Hooker, R., Tucker, T., Tanna, N. and Honnor, S. (2004) Health and the Internet: changing boundaries in primary care, *Family Practice*, 21: 189–91.

Manias, E., Aitken, R. and Dunning, T. (2005) Graduate nurses' communication with health professionals when managing patients' medications, *Journal of Clinical Nursing*, 14: 354–62.

Marvel, M.K., Epstein, R.M., Flowers, K. and Beckman, H.B. (1999) Soliciting the patient's agenda: have we improved? *Journal of the American Medical Association*, 281: 283–7.

Miller, P. and Rose, N. (1994) On therapeutic authority: psychoanalytical expertise under advanced liberalism, *History of the Human Sciences*, 7(3): 29–64.

Nielsen, D.M., Gill, K. and Ricketts, D.M. (2005) Satisfaction levels in orthopaedic outpatients, *Annals of the Royal College of Surgeons of England*, 87: 106–8.

Nettleton, S. and Burrows, R. (2003) E-scaped medicine? Information, reflexivity and health, *Critical Social Policy*, 23(2): 165–85.

Newnes, C. and Radcliffe, N. (2005) *Making and Breaking Children's Lives*. Ross on Wye: PCCS Books.

Nowotny, H. (1981) Women in public life in Austria, in C.F. Epstein and R.L. Coser (eds) *Access to Power: Cross-national Studies of Women and Elites*. London: George Allen and Unwin.

Office for National Statistics (1999) *Cancer 1971–97* [CD Rom]. London: Office for National Statistics.

Osgood, C.E. (1957) Motivational dynamics of language behavior, in N.M. Jones (ed.) *Nebraska Symposium on Motivation*. Lincoln, NE: University of Nebraska Press.

Potter, J. and Wetherell, M. (1987) *Discourse and Social Psychology: Beyond Attitudes and Behaviour*. London: Sage.

Rogers, E. (2003) *The Diffusion of Innovations*, 5th edn. New York: Simon and Schuster.

Rose, N. (1990) *Governing the Soul*. London: Routledge.

Rutherford, J., Leigh, J., Monk, J. and Murray, C. (2005) Creating an organizational infrastructure to develop and support new nursing roles: a framework for debate, *Journal of Nursing Management*, 13: 97–105.

Sarangi, S. (2004) Towards a communicative mentality in medical and health care practice, *Communication and Medicine*, 1(1): 1–11.

Silverman, J., Kurtz, S. and Draper, J. (1998) *Skills for Communicating with Patients*. Oxford: Radcliffe Medical Press.

Stott, R. (2004) Seven lessons from Africa, *British Medical Journal*, 329: 1193.

Tate, P. (2001) *The Doctor's Communication Handbook*, 3rd edn. Oxford: Radcliffe Medical Press.

Wellman, B. (1997) An electronic group is virtually a social network, in S. Kiesler (ed.) *Cultures of the Internet*. Mahwah, NJ: Lawrence Erlbaum.

Wensing, M., Jung, H.P., Mainz, J., Oleson, F. and Grol, R. (1998) A systematic review of the literature on patient priorities for general practice care. Part 1: description of the research domain, *Social Science and Medicine*, 47(10): 1573–88.

West, P. (2004) *Conspicuous Compassion: Why Sometimes It Really Is Cruel to Be Kind*. London: Institute for the Study of Civil Society.

Wilkinson, S., Roberts, A. and Aldridge, J. (1998) Nurse–patient communication in palliative care: an evaluation of a communication skills programme, *Palliative Medicine*, 12: 13–22.

Wilson, P. (2004) The tabloid fixation on superbugs, *British Medical Journal*, 329: 578.

4   The narratives of illness

Narrating sickness

Illness and illness narratives have been the subject of many books, academic articles and popular journalism over the last 20 years or so, and the narrative 'root metaphor' has appealed to health care practitioners as they struggle to make sense of their clients' suffering. There have been so many studies of illness narrative it would be impossible to review them all in a single chapter but we will sketch the broad outlines of this approach and move on to consider how exactly one can address the question of evidence in this context. A good deal would depend on the kinds of evidence a researcher is looking for. Despite the current popularity of this kind of writing, and the conviction that somehow it must do people some good to tell their story, finding evidence of the kind that would convince a sceptical empiricist would be difficult.

Put crudely, narratives are the stories that people tell about their lives (Gray et al. 2005). As Prince called it, 'the recounting ... of one or more real or fictitious events' (1991: 58). Some would argue this definition is incomplete and that a text should describe at least two events for it to be considered a narrative (Barthes 1982; Rimmon-Kenan 2002). Frid et al. (2000) add the importance of a point of view, and that this is what distinguishes narratives from stories: 'narrative is an account of events experienced by the narrator', while storytelling is 'the repeated telling or reading of a story by persons other than the narrator' (p. 695). Paley and Eva add more:

> What is required, we think, is the sense of one thing leading to another; the idea that something happened as a result of something else (which is absent from the nurse/doctor example above). In saying this, we are agreeing with another group of critics who argue, not only that a narrative must include reference to two or more events, but also that some of those events must be causally related.
>
> (2005: 86)

Narrators render the events of their lives meaningful by linking them to other life events, through links forged between these and the general experience of a broader sweep of humanity, and by providing temporal ordering of these events. Importantly, in the light of the concerns about culture and context we raised in the previous chapter, narratives formulate the context for human activity, which might be temporal, spatial, interpersonal or societal (Clandinin and Connelly 2000). Narratives are almost invariably situated within a broader cultural and social context and some theorists see them as revealing social structures and processes. A narrative may be read as representing particular experiences related to race, social class, gender or the particular historical time when it was formulated, rather than merely rendering personal realities. It has been a mainstay of the narrative approach that people use narratives to construct identities for themselves (Gergen 1991, 2001). Through stories, individuals actively construct identities, revise them, and, of particular interest in therapeutic contexts, try out alternative configurations of self (White and Epston 1989; Bell 1999; Besley 2002). Gray et al. (2005) identify that the particular strength of the narrative approach is that it enables us to ground out analyses in how human beings typically understand and represent their lives. One of the tenets of narrative theory is that the world must be interpreted and given narrative form in order for us to make sense of the temporal nature of life.

Within the now burgeoning literature on narratives in the health care disciplines, narratives are represented as resources both for qualitative research (Frank 2000; Frid et al. 2000; Aranda and Street 2001; McCance et al. 2001) and as a means of understanding and enhancing the clinical relationship itself (Greenhalgh and Hurwitz 1998; Charon and Montello 2002).

The health care disciplines have been particularly adept at drawing on the study of narratives as a means of enquiry. Many of these ideas were developed in other disciplines. Sociology has contributed to numerous aspects of narrative enquiry. Berger and Luckman's (1963) contention that important aspects of shared human realities, including identity itself, were constructed through social processes laid the ground for many further inquiries into how stories structured the world (Maines 1993; Gotham and Staples 1996), especially in the sociology of health and illness (Bochner 2001; Bury 2001). Sociological research in narrative has been propelled especially by a number of landmark texts (Mishler 1986; Polkinghorne 1988; Frank 1995) which helped establish the style, format and epistemological warrant for a narrative-based social science. In psychology, narrative approaches have latterly flourished as a result of the hard work of some early pioneers (Sarbin 1986; Bruner 1991) in the face of the discipline's often self-consciously scientific stance. Scholars have taken an interest in topics such as trauma (Crossley 2000) and memory (Neisser and Fivush 1994), and have been concerned with the acquisition of narrative structures by children (Kemper 1984; Mandler 1984). The narrative interpretation of lifespan development has been explored too (Gergen and Gergen 1986).

All these disciplines have in turn drawn on literary criticism and linguistics which have yielded a vast literature on narrative and narratology (Labov and Walentzky 1967; Chatman 1978; Genette 1980; Bakhtin 1981; Toolan 2001; Rimmon-Kenan 2002).

In connection with all these currents in the social and human sciences, then, a narrative approach has increasingly been used to study illness experience, as well as the experience of carers and practitioners of various kinds (e.g. Murray and McMillan 1988; Frank 1995; Bell 1999; Ezzy 2000). Illness was seen as a kind of 'biographical disruption' by Bury (1982) which presented challenges to individuals to re-imagine, re-story and re-tell their life narratives. Studying the 'illness narratives' of sick people thus reveals how illness gets integrated into people's lives and how various psychosocial factors inform this process.

As Gray et al. (2005) remark, the narrative approach, while increasingly embraced by the other social sciences, has been slow to take root in health psychology, perhaps because the latter has its origins in a biomedical model and erstwhile reliance theories which saw health behaviour as resulting from cognitive and attitudinal factors which could be measured quantitatively (Radley 1999). This has meant that traditional health psychology has hitherto not been well equipped to address the perspectives of ill people (Gray et al. 2005). Critical, narrative-oriented scholars have asserted that attempting to quantify aspects of experience is an overly crude way to capture the expressive quality of being ill, and the complex, pervasive 'world of illness' (Radley 1993). While qualitative methods are better able to investigate such complexities, proponents of narrative approaches contend that some qualitative approaches tend to fragment the accounts of the people they study. Abstracting pieces of discourse from their social and temporal context (Murray 1999) is contrasted with narrative approaches with an emphasis on preserving rather than dismembering the stories that are told, which as Gray et al. (2005) suggest, makes the study of health care 'more relevant to the actual lives of ill people'.

Narratives and health professionals

The last couple of decades have seen a growing interest in the experiences and narratives of health professionals, in terms of their socialization and professionalization, their accumulating clinical experience, their own experiences with illness as they struggle to provide services for others and even the reflections they have at the end of their lives. This has arisen partly in response to the concern that the training of health professionals, especially doctors, has emphasized the acquisition of biomedical knowledge at the expense of creating a broadminded, mature, reflective individual.

Over the years, a number of educators have attempted to remedy this situation by exploiting the interdependency of literature and medicine (Hawkins and McEntyre 2000; Das Gupta 2003) as well as the inherently narrative structure of patient histories. Using literature to teach trainee physicians is becoming an increasingly widespread practice, especially in the USA, which, when it works well, can yield benefits in terms of increased empathy, greater understanding of the ethical dimensions of the physician's role, and what has been called 'narrative knowledge', that is, empathy gained through the study of literature and the structure of narrative (Charon et al. 1995).

Personal illness narratives differ from other writing exercises utilized in medical training, including 'critical incident reports' and clinical journal writing or clinically based reflection, in that they do not describe clinical scenarios in which the student is on the doctor side of the doctor–patient relationship (Branch et al. 1993; Patterson 1995; Wong et al. 1995). They share more similarity to writing exercises that rely upon the student physician making an empathic shift in perspective. For instance, exercises in which students compose letters to their early physical examination patients or write autobiographical sketches of their gross anatomy cadavers rely upon the students' ability to step beyond the solely medical perspective (e.g. Reifler 1996). In addition, exercises in writing a clinical story from the patient's point of view or rewriting a patient's narrative from a first-person perspective encourage students to reduce the emotional distance between self and patient (Marshall and O'Keeffe 1995).

There has recently been a renewed interest in the idea of a 'wounded healer' (Jackson 2001). While this may refer to members of the caring professions who have become ill themselves, or might refer to those who have become victims of 'stress' or 'burnout', Jackson argues that it may refer in a much more general sense to the inner 'woundedness' of a healer – their own suffering and vulnerability, which might contribute crucially to the capacity to heal. It may be, says Jackson, that for many healers there are lingering effects left upon them from their personal experiences of illness. These may include lessons learned that may appear bewildering at the time but later serve a constructive purpose, perhaps in the form of attitudes and sensitivities they might draw upon in treating their patients, or perhaps as symptoms or characteristics that usefully influence their therapeutic activities. Thus, their own experiences as sufferers may enhance their healing capacities. Indeed, some reflective writers on the processes involved in healing have warned against the detached professionalism which characterizes many caring disciplines (Brandon 1999).

As Wear and Aultman (2005: 1058) add, the basic tenet linking narrative to medicine is that we can learn a great deal about doctors' and patients' lives by reading and interpreting literary texts; by carefully attending to the stories patients and their families tell; and by 'writing about oneself and one's struggles, about relationships formed with patients, or about patients themselves'.

This venerable interrelationship between storytelling and medicine has found its way, as we have observed, into curricula for medical students, and the ideal of narrative has recently played an increasingly substantial role in the medical humanities in the Americas, as well as Europe and Asia, as a recent issue of the journal *Academic Medicine* has shown (Dittrich 2003). Indeed, narrative and derivatives such as narrative medicine, narrative-based medicine and narrative bioethics have gained a foothold in many medical establishments and in research and curriculum development throughout the world (Charon 2001, 2004).

Sometimes, of course, the use of narratives, stories and anecdotes in the education of health professionals is less successful. Wear and Aultman (2005) describe a course which drew heavily on *The Color Purple* (Walker 1982) in attempting to get students to think about issues such as family structure and poverty. The students were unimpressed, preferring instead, presumably, accounts of poverty which emphasize individual culpability, and not recognizing the legitimacy of the extended family structure that eventually develops around the central character in the novel, Celie. Sometimes then, it is difficult to recognize oneself as implicated in the social forces that create the climate of obstacles the other must confront (Boler 1999: 159). If students and colleagues can be tempted into consideration of their role in larger scale social processes and divisions, then this can contribute to an education that does more than merely add knowledge. It may change the way participants think in a process that Boler (1999) calls the 'pedagogy of discomfort' which involves educators and students in critical enquiry regarding their own values and beliefs, and to examine the relationship between how one perceives others' and one's own constructed self-images. The process focuses on the way emotions define how and what one chooses to see and, conversely, not to see. This enquiry is best undertaken as a collective rather than an individualized process (Boler 1999: 177–8; Wear and Aultman 2005) and the puzzle facing educators is how this may be made possible in classrooms of increasingly middle-class youngsters seeking to enter the health professions.

The narratives of illness: from patients to storytellers

The role of patients' narratives in medicine is a long and illustrious one (Bury 2001). Prior to the popularization of nineteenth-century 'bio-medical models' of illness in the way disease was conceptualized, the role of the doctor in taking a history from the patient was paramount. It often involved considerably more than physical symptoms. It might, as Bury (2001) remarks, involve information about the patient's lifestyle, his or her moral stance and the patient's wider familial or social environment. Elite doctors treating patients from the upper classes in the seventeenth and eighteenth centuries were unlikely to perform a very thorough or detailed physical examination of the patient. Instead, it was considered more appropriate to attend to patients' narratives and adapt treatment regimens to the particular case in hand, usually through procedures that restored the body's equilibrium (Lawrence 1994: 12) deriving from much earlier Hippocratic ideas concerning the balance between the four 'humours'. Such procedures, including bleeding, purging and cupping, have mainly fallen into disuse, with the possible exception of administering laxatives, which still remains popular. By contemporary standards they are not deemed to be efficacious, but presumably by the criteria of the time they were considered worthwhile. Surgery was not considered an appropriate craft for a gentleman. Thus, as Roy Porter put it: 'In the absence of decisive anatomical or physiological expertise, and without a powerful arsenal of cures and surgical skills, the ability to diagnose and make prognoses was highly valued, and an intimate physician–patient relationship was fostered' (1997: 9–10)

The domination of practical medicine by biomedical ideas, images and technologies was, however, never complete. In the mid-twentieth century vociferous practitioners like Balint (1957) kept alive the notion that it was desirable to talk to patients. Towards the end of the twentieth century an increasing body of scholars, spearheaded by some who were also medically trained physicians, reinstated the role of narrative study as an important part of the health care disciplines. As Arthur Kleinman argued, in the face of chronic illness especially, the physician may be best employed as a witness to suffering and to act as a source of practical advice and guidance, based on the 'sensitive solicitation of the patient's and the family's stories of the illness' (1988: 10). As Bury (2001) notes, this renewed attention to patients' narratives suggests that practitioners might be redefining their roles away from a preoccupation with a reductionist bio-medical model of illness.

As we have seen in the previous chapter, there are some features of this expansion of interest of medicine into these socio-emotional territories which deserve further analysis (Bury 2001) and which might involve a subtle re-engineering of the client and the health professional in line with the new narrative-oriented ethos.

The nature of narratives means that they are uniquely suited to the investigation of illness experience. The sick person who tells these kinds of tales provides the researcher and practitioner with two distinct yet related kinds of information (Bury 2001). First, the exploration of chronic illness narratives may throw light on the feelings and meanings attached to the disrupted experience, and the actions, both collective and individual, which are taken to deal with it. Second, the study of illness narratives can potentially reveal the role of a broader suite of important issues, illuminating links between identity, experience and contemporary cultures. Thus, while they are individual in nature, often idiosyncratically so, illness narratives are taken to reveal grander social phenomena, and presumably inform researchers and sensitize practitioners to their meanings.

Bury (2001) identifies two facets of illness narrative. They may be contingent – that is, concerned with beliefs and knowledge about the nature of the illness; and they may also be moral – that is, involving an evaluative dimension concerning the relationship between the individual and their social world and how it might have been changed by illness.

This contingent unfolding of difficulties in illness stories is reflected in some of our own data. There are often many interconnected facets to the experience of illness, all appearing to be mutually interdependent. Moreover, illnesses are often experiences with a history, sometimes going back before the person could reasonably be expected to remember. Here is a middle-aged participant talking about her illness experience to our colleague, Vicky Roberts ('I' for 'interviewer'), as part of a project looking at the experience of long-term ill health:

I: Perhaps erm, is there anything about your erm, your health at this present time that impacts upon your life in any way?

R: I suffer from arthritis in my face, neck and spine. I did have an operation, erm, a few years ago, erm, 18 years ago on my left side of my face and they found nobules [sic], arthritic nobules, and they were going again to operate on these. What I've basically got is I've got no cartilage on one side, and very thin cartilage on the other side, so it rubs a lot. So I suffer very badly from headaches ... but they could come from the arthritis or from ... so I can never tell. I mean I've tried acupuncture and I can't cope with it. I think I'm about the only person who can't! Erm, it just sends me doo-lally. But it ... I'm just so sensitive to pain that she had to stop. I had more pain with acupuncture than I did without. I've tried everything! I mean at the moment I'm going to back class to try and stop this pain in my back, which today is horrendous, and I don't know where that's come from! Erm, it ... I don't take medication. So I basically not so much prefer the pain but, erm (pause), I don't know how to explain it. I'm not, I'm not, I won't take medication because, well, I don't believe in medication. I will take it if I'm like today. I had to take a tablet because I just couldn't cope with the back, although my face at the moment is very painful. It only affects me in as much as it affects my temperament sometimes. I can be a bit irritated because I try and override the pain. Sometimes I can't walk very far, I have a, I have a blue badge on the basis that one of the question [sic] is how far can you walk before any/before you have any com ... erm, discomfort or pain, and I can't. So my answer was no I can't, cos I'm in constant discomfort and pain all the time. Some days are definitely better than other days. When I was at the caravan for the two weeks I came back and I felt better. This week has been quite bad, so it varies. I certainly feel that since I've been going to back class the person told me that he could tell the difference it's about 50 minutes of different exercises and they vary it every week you go. And he said, you definitely become more supple but you just can't get rid of the pain, and you can't understand why if I bend down, I can't get back up again if I can walk alright. The pain … so he doesn't know where it's coming from. And you're a bit sort of like, no I can't understand it. I said sometimes my body feels as if it is a 90-year-old body.

I: So it's quite a consistent feature of your life then?

R: It has been for the last … the back problem is definitely for the last 6 months, erm (pause) my face, my mother said, up to a year old I was fine (pause) well after I had my first birthday I suffered very much from earaches.

I: OK.

We have quoted this participant at some length so as to highlight the complexities of the illness narrative. We can see here the oscillation between medical details of the most incredible precision, relating to the quality of cartilage, to the radical imprecision of 'this pain in my back' – 'I don't know where that's come from'. An important feature here, in our experience characteristic of accounts of low-level ill health, is the diversity of symptomatology that does not neatly fit a single category but which is meticulously partitioned by the sufferer into different areas of distress, where the arthritis is distinguished from the back pain. There are causal theories proposed for different aspects of the problems, from the headaches being related to the arthritic nodules or 'nobules' and the cartilage, yet there are other areas of radical indeterminacy, such as the pains that have remained enigmatic to the exercise class instructor. This quotation has been included in its entirety, rather than analytically separating out different aspects, so as to give a sense of the apparent chaos which assails the listener or reader. Arthur Frank (1995) identifies three kinds of illness narrative, the 'restitution narrative', the 'chaos narrative' and the 'quest narrative'. Of these, the foregoing account perhaps most closely resembles the 'chaos narrative'. Often, these chaos narratives remain submerged, and the apparent lack of coherence may reflect the individual having been overwhelmed by the intensity of their illness.

At the same time, in this account we see some attempt to tentatively stand outside the chaos so that the story can begin to emerge. Frank (1995: 98) calls it 'the anti-narrative of time without sequence, telling without mediation and speaking about oneself without being fully able to reflect on oneself'. To Frank, chaos narratives are often disjointed and without sequence, containing an underlying message that life does not get better. In the example quoted earlier there are some signals of attempts to do without medication for example, yet the enormity of the task, compounded by the inexplicable bad back has driven the teller back to taking a tablet. As Frank describes it, the chaos narrative involves anxiety, human frailty and vulnerability. In Frank's view, revealing how easily each of us could be toppled has a deep effect on the listener.

By contrast, in the West, says Frank, we are mainly preoccupied with the 'restitution narrative', which goes: 'Yesterday I was healthy, today I am sick but tomorrow I will be healthy again'. There is a belief that the person can be restored to health. Where illness and disability are chronic the person's experience does not fit this model and so they can find it *difficult* to tell a story which does *not* appear to have a happy ending.

The third form of illness story identified by Frank (1995) is the quest narrative, in which a person journeys through and faces suffering in the belief that something is to be gained or somehow sense can be made from the illness experience. Quest stories search for meaning, patterns, regularities or ways of managing the condition. In a sense they represent the sufferer looking for alternative ways of being ill, or even alternative ways of being well. Returning to our informant then, we discover that she has a suite of illnesses that extend considerably beyond the merely chaotic. Where her 'food intoleration' is concerned she is able to place the experience in a more meaningful framework and thus at least partially to bring it under some measure of subjective control:

I: So is that what it feels like then? Almost like a battle between yourself and this pain?

R: Yes because sometimes I get so depressed I sometimes wonder, what, what's the point? Because with me, with my food intoleration as well. When, when you, I mean you know, er everybody, we're all the same particularly us women, if we go on a diet and we're going to, we're going to er alright, we're not gonna have the chocolate, we're not going to have that cake, we're gonna have a little bit less food. [pause] You crave it more.

I: Yeah!

R: And my food, if I eat certain things, will affect me, will effect [sic] my, erm, metabolism, and I'm on the toilet for 15 minutes with cramps. So I try not to eat that food, but sometimes I crave that.

I: So you've got quite a few . . .

R: So, so wanting something, and then with the pains, and you think, well you can't eat that because you know what will happen. And I was lucky yesterday with that rich food cos I thought, I'm gonna suffer, but I didn't and I was really pleased. Erm and yet I'll have a yogurt drink which doesn't affect me during the day, and I'll have it at night and yet I'm on the flippin' thing for 15 minutes. And because of that, and I have to watch exactly what I'm eating, and the only thing I really miss I suppose is bread, cos I used to like fresh loaves and that . . . I'm not too keen on sliced bread, but the walnut loaves and things like that I would like, so I miss that. Erm, and because I think, oh I would have that piece of cake, but what's in it, you know.

I: So have you got quite a few food intolerances then?

R: Erm, I'm intolerant to wheat, and dairy products so like mayonnaise sauces, white sauces, anything like that, which is what I had yesterday with cheese as well. I've also got bilirubin, which is, er my liver doesn't act . . . it's a very common thing apparently. But my liver acts slower, so therefore I can't eat fried food, I can't eat anything with yeast, erm, anything like those packet soups. In fact, last year at camp, the Polish did a barsh, and they used one of their packet soups, which is about as bad as our packet soups, it's got all sorts of rubbish in it. And, it's never happened before to me, and mum's . . . I'm sitting by my mother I'm doing this, and my mother's saying, 'what on earth are you scratching for'. I said, 'I'm itching' and she said, '[participant's name], look at yourself'. And this stuff had made me come out in a rash, on my arms, my face and my and my, erm, my torso at the top. And I'd come out that fast!

Here we have a theorization of the plight which is altogether more coherent than the earlier part of the story concerning arthritis and bad backs. Here we have system and order, a more or less moral universe where food is classifiable according to its propensity to make one ill and, with the precision of a religious devotee, the quantities and the times at which the supplicant is allowed it are meticulously spelled out. If this regimen is departed from, then the expected worsening of one's health is feared, and the lack of this, far from indicating the capricious and random nature of the symptoms, is interpreted in juridical terms, as if one had got away with something or escaped the consequences of a natural law.

In a paper by Williams (1993), this theme of morality in chronic illness is expanded. Patients' stories are located within a cultural framework within which health is portrayed as a virtuous state. Although 'illness' may no longer be regarded as having a close connection with sin (p. 92), the kinds of regime to which our participant subscribes recollect the view that much illness results from 'inappropriate' individual behaviours, and a morally recognizable regime of foodstuffs, with some items meriting restriction, or even being 'rubbish', the indulgence in which is responsible for the illness. This is reminiscent of how Williams describes 'coping strategies' designed to maximize the sufferer's ability to engage in normal activities, 'revealed a vulnerability and a sense of urgency' which amounted to the 'pursuit of virtue' (p. 96).

In Frank's (1995, 1997) seminal work, now over a decade old, which draws upon both his own biographical experience and other people's autobiographical narratives there is further evidence of the 'moral' aspect of illness narratives in Bury's (2001) sense of the term. Seeing the growing raft of people who live with persistent health problems, Frank talks of a 'remission society', where people live with chronic disorders, or in states of 'recovery' that never quite amount to cure. Frank suggests that we may speak of people trying to be 'successfully ill' in such contexts (1997: 117). Even more significantly, he suggests that illness and suffering present people with a 'moral opening for witness and change' (p. 141). As we can see in the earlier examples, illness presents an opportunity for progressively carving out new dimensions of selfhood. The ongoing experience of illness, and the sometimes fraught encounters with health care professionals it entails, enable sufferers to identify more clearly their own personal values. Under conditions of adversity, some of which are furnished by the health professions themselves, people may grasp illness 'as an active responsibility first to understand the self, and then to place the self within an extensive ecology of relationships' (p. 142). This may be, as seen earlier, the relationships with other family members or it might involve those in wider society. Within the experience of illness, people may attempt to rescue some valued aspects of life, against the onslaught of symptoms and their effects on self and others. As Charmaz has put it: 'chronic illness often crystallizes vital lessons about living' (1991: vii).

Critical notice: the limits of narrative

Of course, a movement as large and diverse as that seeking a knowledge of the narratives of practitioners and clients will not be without its critics. At this time, it is relatively rare to hear criticism of the approach *per se*, but there are arguments going on concerning the appropriate way to proceed and the meanings that can be deduced from the narrative data which are rapidly accumulating.

Paley and Eva (2005) identify several different schools of thought within narrative theory in the social sciences, which they urge us to treat with some degree of scepticism because of the all too glib elision between a number of important distinctions for example stories and the reality they seek to describe or narratives and the experiences and cognitions which allegedly underlie them. Any attempt to bring the ideas of narratives into the realm of evidence-based practice must take these ideas seriously because it is necessary to be clear as to just what exactly a narrative is and what it is trying to describe. Paley and Eva's typology is necessarily slightly exaggerated but they do this in order to highlight what they see to be the folly of some of these positions:

1. *Naïve realism* The first tendency is for authors to take narratives as if they were reliable reports. For example, 'personal accounts are taken only at face value' (Bury 2001: 281; McAllister 2001). Paley and Eva call this 'naïve realism' as applied to narrative, where the story told is treated as if it were unproblematically a record of 'what happened'. If pushed on the point, of course, most writers probably wouldn't claim to believe this in a strong form, but in practice when research is being written up for publication the participant's account is frequently taken as authoritative (Chambers 1998; Dunniece and Slevin 2000; Frid et al. 2000).

2. *What it means to the teller of the tale* The second premise that infuses a good deal of work in the field of narrative enquiry is that a narrative represents 'what it means to the teller of the tale' (Blumenfeld-Jones 1995: 26), reveals the 'truth of personal experience' (Sakalys 2000), and provides 'access to an authentic self' (Taylor 2003: 250). In this view, the thorny question of truth is bracketed off and instead of focusing on the question of 'how it was' researchers concentrate on 'how it seems to me' (Leight 2002). In this genre of research, writers are less concerned with truth in an absolute sense and more concerned with 'meaning', the subject's perception, not whether that perception corresponds with 'reality' (Launer 1998; Bailey and Tilley 2002).

3. *Narrative is intrinsically fictional* This idea can be traced back to Sartre (1965) who believed that there are no true stories, and has proved popular with postmodernist historians (White 1987; Hutcheon 1988; Jenkins 1995). However, this assumption can also be detected in health care literature: 'all narratives are socially constructed and thus, forms of fictions' (Crawford et al. 1995 Aranda and Street 2001: 792). However, this 'does not invalidate them for research purposes', because stories 'can achieve a degree of critical

significance ... and promote emancipatory moments' (Barone 1995: 64; Blumenreich 2004).

4. *Narrative is a mode of explanation* This idea was strongly promoted in psychology by Bruner (1985), who originally argued that narrative is a type of cognition which differs from 'paradigmatic' (scientific) cognition. Narratives explain phenomena by referring to 'the particular and special characteristics of each action' (Polkinghorne 1995: 11), whereas scientific explanations refer to what is common to a class of actions. This kind of approach can be seen in McCance et al.'s (2001) study of the perceived meaning of caring.

Furthermore, there are other critical positions that argue against the notion that we can use narratives in any naïve realist sense to explore what happened, what events mean to the person, or what kinds of cognitive, interpretive practices they are using to 'make sense' of the phenomena in question. This view tends to see the 'subject' or the person as somehow pre-existing the narratives or discourses which they are using to undertake this sense-making process. A more radical suggestion, present in a good many of the founding texts of this narrative movement, is to pose the problem the other way around. The individual, including the sense of self, the experience of consciousness and the interpretations they make can be seen as the products of discourse. As Nelson and McGillion (2004) describe, the view that discourses actively construct these senses of self or, as they have been called, 'subject-positions' has important implications for the theories of the self that accompany the narrative turn in social science and health studies. These more radical accounts of the representation and constitution of the self build upon Foucault (1986, 1987) and Giddens (1990), and proceed from the assumption that subjectivity is not an existing 'thing' but a process – a discursively constructed way of being. In this framework, the sense of being an individual subject comes about through the operation of power relationships and societal processes and forces which are not necessarily visible to the individuals so constituted in a direct and obvious way. Our very selves, then, are a product or function of unseen societal and political power, 'which requires us to behave in particular ways and to be a certain type of person' (Nelson and McGillion 2004: 632–3).

In his *Discipline and Punish*, Michel Foucault (1995) analyses how European governments learned over the past few centuries that rather than control their citizenry by violence and terror, it was more efficient to use more subtle kinds of discipline, which operated through examination, observation and record-keeping. This eventually becomes internalized by individuals themselves. Christopher Lasch (1985) describes a similar process in his analysis of the 'tutelary complex', and David Smail (2005) analyses how we turn our attention inward in a kind of anxious self-monitoring, keeping us perpetually comparing our 'selves' with others. The saturation of the early twenty-first-century news and entertainment media with material pertaining to 'celebrities'; the creation of a media industry built to uphold neo-liberal business-friendly ideologies, where it is these ideologies that matter, not their creatures. Rather than originating with the individual celebrity, 'charisma' is instead the visible aspect of a power which is temporarily accorded him or her by the media world. It can, of course, be instantly withdrawn and the star eclipsed once new and potentially more lucrative disportations present themselves. This kind of spectacle, says Smail (2005), reinforces the notion that our personal worth is based on the individual exercise of our interior powers.

Rather than representing unmediated access to the individual's interpretations, cognitions or sense of identity, in this view narratives emerge from a process of what Foucault termed 'self-fashioning'. Nelson and McGillion (2004) argue that understanding this is vital to making sense of the way in which subjectivity and discourse together create the 'subject' of narrative research. In Foucault's notion of governmentality, there is a 'circular process' (Minson 1993) whereby this constellation of practices – discursively constructed and 'freely' chosen – produces advanced liberalism's modern humanist subject (Foucault 1991; Rose 1999). This then, in a roundabout way, helps explain why our narratives look and feel the way they do. How, despite feeling intensely personal, they are full of recognizable structures, processes, events, characters and even literary motifs.

This is not to say that the accounts provided by health care workers are in a deceptive sense inauthentic, and no doubt they represent the firsthand perspective on expertise entertained by the practitioners themselves. Nor do we wish to refute narrative as a worthwhile method for providing an account of practice. However, as Smail (2005) argues, rather than being a behaviour-causing, narrative-creating schema, localizable inside people's heads, the self, its expertise, powers of will, and its associated 'narratives' can best be understood as social or discursive constructions, distributed throughout a network which extends far beyond the individual who appears to host them.

The concern over the use of narratives in research on health care and therapy goes even further in some quarters. Paul Atkinson and David Silverman (Atkinson 1997; Atkinson and Silverman 1997) contend that social scientists need to be story analysts and not storytellers. They express strong reservations about the narrative turn in social science, calling it 'a blind alley', a 'preoccupation with the revelation of personal experience through confession and therapeutic discourse', 'a vulgar realism', and 'hyperauthentic', 'misleading', 'sentimental', 'exaggerated', naïvely 'heroic', and representing a 'romantic construction of the self'. Atkinson and Silverman do not renounce all narrative research, and have engaged in some of their own (Pithouse and Atkinson 1988; Atkinson 1994). They are disquieted by personal, autobiographical and illness narratives, especially where they can see no analysis, and the narratives are not treated as a social phenomenon which tell us something about the social context within which they are produced and understood, and presented without what they see to be appropriate methodological skepticism.

Conclusion: towards evidence-based narrative

Finally, it is appropriate after the intoxicating journey through the study of illness and narrative, to pause once again and examine its relationship to the theme of our book – evidence-based health communication. Evidence-based practice and narrative practice are often seen as incompatible perspectives (Taylor 2003). As Taylor reminds us, the ethos of evidence-based practice is to resolutely assert the primacy of scientifically derived knowledge. This is a particular form of knowledge, in which propositional content (knowing that) dominates, and where as we have described, the cumulative evidence from experimentally based activities is privileged. In some health care disciplines, especially nursing, other forms of making sense of the natural and phenomenal world have been popular, particularly the notion of reflective practice. This takes issue with the assumption in evidence-based practice approaches that positivist knowledge can be applied directly to practice situations. Here, the work of Donald Schön (e.g. 1983) is often drawn upon to provide a theoretical grounding for reflective practice. Schön has become positioned as one of the key exponents of an alternative to a 'technical-rational' approach to professional practice. Schön famously made a distinction between what he called the 'high hard ground' where 'manageable problems lend themselves to solution through the application of research-based theory and technique' and the swampy lowlands where 'messy, confusing problems defy technical solution' (1987: 3).

In line with these formulations of the issue of how evidence may be applied to practical matters, Ban (2003: 75) has argued that 'one aspect of EBM that receives comparatively little attention is that genuine evidence-based practice presupposes an *interpretive paradigm*, within which the patient experiences illness and the clinician–patient encounter is enacted'. Some have argued that there is a politics of evidence at work in health care so that activities which are language based, client directed and focused on relational processes are difficult to incorporate in evidence-based medicine (Larner 2004). Yet the narratives of illness often reveal a good deal about how people formulate their identities and their problems and are also an important source of understanding when it comes to cultural diversities and intercultural interpretation. The purpose of this chapter is not merely to rehearse the well-known criticisms of a strong evidence-based practice approach, but to argue for a rapprochement between the two different traditions, and explore the work which is beginning to address the effects of narratives in health care. Taylor (2003) adds that both narrative approaches to health care and conventional scientific medicine are themselves narrative forms so they both will repay critical scrutiny. The human stories we tell one another, just as much as the scientific accounts, are artfully constructed.

The broad concepts of language underlying many of the narrative approaches to health care studies are indebted to Wittgenstein (1953). The premise of Wittgenstein's philosophical investigations is that meaning is not merely *found* in the world in any simple sense; meaning making is an activity through which people make and give meaning to what they encounter. As one of the slogans of Wittgensteinian scholars had it, 'the meaning is the use'. From Wittgenstein's point of view, language exists within a culture and is based on public 'agreements-in-practice', criteria or rules. These rules cannot be learnt explicitly, but are related to the deep cultural agreement or 'doxa' that forms the background against which narratives make sense. In this view, we become socialized into a language as we are socialized into the culture within which it exists. Thus, by the time we become aware of it we cannot just assign any meaning to language as we see fit, like Lewis Carroll's Humpty Dumpty. The way that narrative analysis explores meaning and how it might offer an emancipatory approach to clients and practitioners positions it in opposition to many systems and biologically based or psychologically grounded theories that assume that some underlying struc-ture or dysfunction determines behaviour (Besley 2002).

Narrative approaches in health care encourage us to reflect on just what it is that our evidence means. To suggest that narratives lack scientific credibility is not to say that they simply didn't happen. In a sense they are most richly evidenced because they are all around us. Talking about one's health, or that of other people is an enormously popular activity. However, it is important to be aware of what the narratives give us evidence of. They don't necessarily give us access directly to processes of sense making, consciousness or mindedness on the part of the narrator, as Paley and Eva (2005) remind us. Neither particularly do they give us direct knowledge of the social context in which the events in the story took place. In a sense, despite their popularity we can make only quite modest claims about the evidence which narratives can provide. However, their role in enriching the picture of health and illness, their potential in enhancing understanding between practitioners and sufferers, their role in educating practitioners and their ability to build solidarity between sufferers themselves cannot be denied. The burgeoning fields of narrative medicine, and the medical humanities are testament to the desire to know something more than can be assessed simply through a symptom checklist or an investigation of the vital signs. As Widder puts it: 'medical humanities are not just a nice side dish of true medicine, but they are an indispensable part of patient oriented medicine' (2004: 103).

References

Aranda, S. and Street, A. (2001) From individual to group: use of narratives in a participatory research process, *Journal of Advanced Nursing*, 33: 791–7.

Atkinson, P. (1994) Rhetoric as skill, in M. Bloor and P. Taraborrelli (eds) *Qualitative Research in Health and Medicine*. Aldershot: Avebury.

Atkinson, P. (1997) Narrative turn or blind alley? *Qualitative Health Research*, 7: 325–44.

Atkinson, P. and Silverman, D. (1997) Kundera's *Immortality*: The interview society and the invention of the self, *Qualitative Inquiry*, 3: 304–25.

Bailey, P.H. and Tilley, S. (2002) Storytelling and the interpretation of meaning in qualitative research, *Journal of Advanced Nursing*, 38: 574–83.

Bakhtin, M.M. (1981) *The Dialogic Imagination* (translated by C. Emerson and M. Holquist). New York: University of Texas Press.

Balint, M. (1957) *The Doctor, His Patient and the Illness*, 2nd edn. London: Pitman Medical.

Ban, N. (2003) Continuing care of chronic illness: evidence-based medicine and narrative-based medicine as competencies for patient-centered care, *Asia Pacific Family Medicine*, 2: 74–6.

Barone, T. (1995) Persuasive writings, vigilant readings, and reconstructed characters: the paradox of trust in educational story sharing, in J.A. Hatch and R. Wisniewski (eds) *Life History and Narrative*. London: Falmer Press.

Barthes, R. (1982) Introduction to the structural analysis of narratives, in S. Sontag (ed.) *A Barthes Reader*. New York: Hill and Wang.

Bell, S.E. (1999) Narratives and lives: women's health politics and the diagnosis of cancer for DES daughters, *Narrative Inquiry*, 9: 347–89.

Berger, P.L. and Luckmann, T. (1963) *The Social Construction of Reality: A Treatise in the Sociology of Knowledge*. Garden City, NY: Doubleday.

Besley, A.C. (2002) Foucault and the turn to narrative therapy, *British Journal of Guidance and Counselling*, 30(2): 125–43.

Blumenfeld-Jones, D. (1995) Fidelity as a criterion for practicing and evaluating narrative enquiry, in J.A. Hatch and R. Wisniewski (eds) *Life History and Narrative*. London: Falmer Press.

Blumenreich, M. (2004) Avoiding the pitfalls of 'conventional' narrative research: using post structural theory to guide the creation of narratives of children with HIV, *Qualitative Research*, 4: 77–90.

Bochner, A.P. (2001) Narrative's virtues, *Qualitative Inquiry*, 7: 131–57.

Boler, M. (1999) *Feeling Power: Emotions and Education*. New York: Routledge.

Branch, W., Pels, R.J., Lawrence, R.S. and Arky, R. (1993) Becoming doctors: critical incident reports from third year medical students, *New England Journal of Medicine*, 329: 1130–2.

Brandon, D. (1999) Melting straitjackets, *Journal of Psychiatric and Mental Health Nursing*, 6: 321–6.

Bruner, J. (1985) *Actual Minds, Possible Worlds*. Cambridge, MA: Harvard University Press.

Bruner, J. (1991) The narrative construction of reality, *Critical Inquiry*, 18: 1–21.

Bury, M. (1982) Chronic illness as biographical disruption, *Sociology of Health and Illness*, 4: 167–82.

Bury, M. (2001) Illness narratives: fact or fiction? *Sociology of Health and Illness*, 23: 263–85.

Chambers, N. (1998) 'We have to put up with it – don't we?' The experience of being the registered nurse on duty, managing a violent incident involving an elderly patient: a phenomenological study, *Journal of Advanced Nursing*, 27: 429–36.

Charmaz, K. (1991) *Good Days, Bad Days: The Self in Chronic Illness and Time*. New Brunswick, NJ: Rutgers University Press.

Charon, R. (2001) Narrative medicine: form, function and ethics, *Annals of Internal Medicine*, 134: 83–7.

Charon, R. (2004) Narrative and medicine, *New England Journal of Medicine*, 350: 862–4.

Charon, R. and Montello, M. (eds) (2002) *Stories Matter: The Role of Narrative in Medical Ethics*. New York: Routledge.

Charon, R., Trautmann Banks, J., Connelly, J.E. et al. (1995) Literature and medicine: contributions to clinical practice, *Annals of Internal Medicine*, 122: 599–606.

Chatman, S. (1978) *Story and Discourse: Narrative Structure in Fiction and Film*. Ithaca, NY: Cornell University Press.

Clandinin, D.J. and Connelly, F.M. (2000) *Narrative Inquiry: Experience and Story in Qualitative Research*. San Francisco, CA: Jossey-Bass.

Crawford, P., Nolan, P. and Brown (1995) *Linguistic Entrapment: Medico-Nursing Biographies as Fictions*, Journal of Advanced Nursing, 22 1141–1148

Crossley, M.L. (2000) *Introducing Narrative Psychology: Self, Trauma, and the Construction of Meaning*. Buckingham: Open University Press.

Das Gupta, S. (2003) Reading bodies, writing bodies: self-reflection and cultural criticism in a narrative medicine curriculum, *Literature and Medicine*, 22(2): 241–56.

Dittrich, L.R. (2003) Preface to specal issue on literature in medicine, *Academic Medicine*, 78(10): 951–3.

Dunniece, U. and Slevin, E. (2000) Nurses' experiences of being present with a patient receiving a diagnosis of cancer, *Journal of Advanced Nursing*, 32: 611–18.

Ezzy, D. (2000) Illness narratives: time, hope and HIV, *Social Science and Medicine*, 50: 605–17.

Foucault, M. (1986) *The History of Sexuality: Care of the Self*, Vol. 3 (translated from the French by Robert Hurley). New York: Pantheon Books.

Foucault, M. (1987) The ethic of the care of self as a practice of freedom, *Philosophy and Social Criticism*, 2(3): 121–31.

Foucault, M. (1991) Governmentality, in G. Burchell, C. Gordon and P. Miller (eds) *The Foucault Effect: Studies in Governmentality*. Chicago: University of Chicago Press.

Foucault, M. (1995) *Discipline and Punish*. New York: Vintage Books.

Frank, A. (1995) *The Wounded Storyteller: Body, Illness, and Ethics*. Chicago: University of Chicago Press.

Frank, A. (1997) Illness as moral occasion: restoring agency to ill people, *Health*, 1(2): 131–48.

Frank, A. (2000) Illness and autobiographical work, *Qualitative Sociology*, 23: 135–56.

Frid, I., Öhlén, J. and Bergbom, I. (2000) On the use of narratives in nursing research, *Journal of Advanced Nursing*, 32: 695–703.

Genette, G. (1980) *Narrative Discourse* (translated by J. Lewin). Ithaca, NY: Cornell University Press.

Gergen, K.J. (1991) *The Saturated Self: Dilemmas of Identity in Contemporary Life*. New York: Basic Books.

Gergen, K.J. (2001). *Social Construction in Context*. London: Sage.

Gergen, K.J. and Gergen, M.M. (1986) Narrative form and the construction of psychological science, in T.R. Sarbin (ed.) *Narrative Psychology: The Storied Nature of Human Conduct*. New York: Praeger.

Giddens, A. (1990) *The Consequences of Modernity*. Cambridge: Polity Press.

Gotham, K.F. and Staples, W.G. (1996) Narrative analysis and the new historical sociology, *Sociological Quarterly*, 37: 481–501.

Gray, R.E., Fergus, K.D. and Fitch, M.I. (2005) Two Black men with prostate cancer: a narrative approach, *British Journal of Health Psychology*, 10: 71–84.

Greenhalgh, T. and Hurwitz, B. (eds) (1998) *Narrative Based Medicine: Dialogue and Discourse in Clinical Practice*. London: BMJ Books.

Hawkins, A.H. and McEntyre, M.C. (2000) *Teaching Literature and Medicine*. New York: MLA Publications.

Hutcheon, L. (1988) *A Poetics of Postmodernism: History, Theory, Fiction*. London: Routledge.

Jackson, S.J. (2001) The wounded healer, *Bulletin of the History of Medicine*, 75: 1–36.

Jenkins, K. (1995) *On 'What Is History?' From Carr and Elton to Rorty and White*. London: Routledge.

Kemper, S. (1984) The development of narrative skills: explanations and entertainments, in S.A. Kuczaj (ed.) *Discourse Development: Progress in Cognitive Development Research*. New York: Springer-Verlag.

Kleinman, A. (1988) *The Illness Narratives: Suffering, Healing and the Human Condition*. New York: Basic Books.

Labov, W. and Walentzky, J. (1967) Narrative analysis: oral versions of personal experience, in J. Helm (ed.) *Essays on the Verbal and Visual Arts*. Seattle, WA: American Ethnological Society.

Larner, G. (2004) Family therapy and the politics of evidence, *Journal of Family Therapy*, 26: 17–39.

Lasch, C. (1985) *The Minimal Self*. London: Picador.

Launer, J. (1998) Narrative and mental health in primary care, in T. Greenhalgh and B. Hurwitz (eds) *Narrative Based Medicine: Dialogue and Discourse in Clinical Practice*. London: BMJ Books.

Lawrence, C. (1994) *Medicine in the Making of Modern Britain 1700–1920*. London: Routledge.

Leight, S.B. (2002) Starry night: using story to inform aesthetic knowing in women's health nursing, *Journal of Advanced Nursing*, 37: 108–14.

McAllister, M.M. (2001) In harm's way: a postmodern narrative inquiry, *Journal of Psychiatric and Mental Health Nursing*, 8: 391–7.

McCance, T.V., McKenna, H.P. and Boore, J.R.P. (2001) Exploring caring using narrative methodology: an analysis of the approach, *Journal of Advanced Nursing*, 33: 350–6.

Maines, D.R. (1993) Narrative's moment and sociology's phenomena: toward a narrative sociology, *Sociological Quarterly*, 34: 17–38.

Mandler, J.M. (1984) *Stories, Scripts and Scenes: Aspects of a Schema Theory*. Hillsdale, NJ: Lawrence Erlbaum Associates.

Marshall, P.A. and O'Keeffe, J.P. (1995) Medical students' first-person narratives of a patient's story of AIDS, *Social Science and Medicine*, 40: 67–76.

Minson J. (1993) *Questions of Conduct: Sexual Harassment, Citizenship, Government*. Houndsmills: Macmillan.

Mishler, E.G. (1986) *Research Interviewing: Context and Narrative*. Cambridge, MA.: Harvard University Press.

Murray, M. (1999) The storied nature of health and illness, in M. Murray and K. Chamberlain (eds) *Qualitative Health Psychology: Theory and Methods*. Thousand Oaks, CA: Sage.

Murray, M. and McMillan, C. (1988) *Working Class Women's View of Cancer*. Belfast: Ulster Cancer Foundation.

Neisser, U. and Fivush, R. (eds) (1994) *The Remembering Self: Construction and Accuracy in the Self-narrative*. New York: Cambridge University Press.

Nelson, S. and McGillion, M. (2004) Expertise or performance? Questioning the rhetoric of contemporary narrative use in nursing, *Journal of Advanced Nursing*, 47(6): 631–8.

Paley, J. and Eva, G. (2005) Narrative vigilance: the analysis of stories in health care, *Nursing Philosophy*, 6: 83–97.

Patterson, B. (1995) Developing and maintaining reflection in clinical journals, *Nurse Education Today*, 15: 211–20.

Pithouse, A. and Atkinson, P. (1988) Telling the case, in N. Coupland (ed.) *English Discourse Styles*. London: Picador.

Polkinghorne, D. (1988) *Narrative Knowing and the Human Sciences*. Albany, NY: State University of New York Press.

Polkinghorne, D. (1995) Narrative configuration in qualitative analysis, in J.A. Hatch and R. Wisniewski (eds) *Life History and Narrative*. London: Falmer Press.

Porter, R. (1997) *The Greatest Benefit to Mankind: A Medical History of Humanity from Antiquity to the Present*. London: Fontana.

Prince, G. (1982) *Narratology: The Form and Functioning of Narrative*. The Hague: Mouton.

Prince, G. (1991) *Dictionary of Narratology*. Aldershot: Scolar Press.

Radley, A. (1993) *Worlds of Illness: Biographical and Cultural Perspectives on Health and Disease*. London: Routledge.

Radley, A. (1999) Social realms and the qualities of illness experience, in M. Murray and K. Chamberlain (eds) *Qualitative Health Psychology: Theory and Methods*. Thousand Oaks, CA: Sage.

Reifler, D.R. (1996) 'I actually don't mind the bone saw': narratives of gross anatomy, *Literature and Medicine*, 15: 183–99.

Rimmon-Kenan, S. (2002) *Narrative Fiction*, 2nd edn. London: Routledge.

Rose, N. (1999) *Governing the Soul: The Shaping of the Private Self*, 2nd edn. London: Routledge.

Sakalys, J.A. (2000) The political role of illness narratives, *Journal of Advanced Nursing*, 31: 1469–75.

Sarbin, T.R. (ed.) (1986) *Narrative Psychology: The Storied Nature of Human Conduct*. New York: Praeger.

Sartre, J.P. (1965) *What Is Literature?* New York: Harper & Row.

Schön, D.A. (1983) *The Reflective Practitioner*. New York: The Free Press.

Schön, D.A. (1987) *Educating the Reflective Practitioner: Towards a New Design for Teaching and Learning in the Professions*. New York: The Free Press.

Smail, D.J. (2005) *Power, Interest and Psychology*: *Elements of a Social Materialist Understanding of Distress*. Ross-on-Wye: PCCS Books.

Taylor, C. (2003) Narrating practice: reflective accounts and the textual construction of reality, *Journal of Advanced Nursing*, 42(3): 244–51.

Toolan, M. (2001) *Narrative: A Critical Linguistic Introduction*, 2nd edn. London: Routledge.

Walker, A. (1982) *The Color Purple*. Orlando, FL: Harcourt.

Wear, D. and Aultman, J.M. (2005) The limits of narrative: medical student resistance to confronting inequality and oppression in literature and beyond, *Medical Education*, 39: 1056–65.

White, H. (1987) *The Content of the Form: Narrative Discourse and Historical Representation*. Baltimore, MD: Johns Hopkins University Press.

White, M. and Epston, D. (1989) *Literate Means to Therapeutic Ends*. Adelaide: Dulwich Centre.

Widder, J. (2004) The origins of medical evidence: communication and experimentation, *Medicine, Health Care and Philosophy*, 7: 99–104.

Williams, G. (1993) Chronic illness and the pursuit of virtue in everyday life, in A. Radley (ed.) *Worlds of Illness: Biographical and Cultural Perspectives on Health and Disease*. London: Routledge.

Wittgenstein, L. (1953) *Philosophical Investigations*, 2nd edn (translated by G.E.M. Anscombe). Oxford: Blackwell.

Wong, F.K.Y., Kember, D., Chung, L.Y.F. and Yan, L. (1995) Assessing the level of student reflection from reflective journals, *Journal of Advanced Nursing*, 22: 48–57.

5 The consultation: towards a 'molecular sociology' of the health care encounter

The past, present and future of consultations

A good deal of health care over the past three millennia has taken place through some sort of face-to-face encounter between a client and an expert; latterly this is usually a health professional in most developed nations. Yet it is only in the last half century that the processes that go on in health care encounters have been studied intensively, since the development of accessible audio and video recording techniques, and more recently computer software that allows large amounts of text to be analysed in seconds. The close attention devoted to interpersonal interaction has been referred to as 'molecular sociology' (Lynch 1993), to denote an even more precise focus than the conventional macro- and micro-sociological approaches to studying the human social world. Consequently, there is a great deal now known about the interactional techniques of health care encounters in clinical settings, especially in the most popular sphere of enquiry, that of doctor–patient interaction. We will explore some of these issues in more detail a little later.

The future of consultations in health care in the UK (and many other nations too) will almost certainly throw up some interesting developments. The creation of large group practices and primary care trusts means that patients are likely to see a whole variety of personnel, not just the familiar GP, thus bringing up a host of questions about the kind and quality of relationships between practitioners and patients and the extent to which an ongoing caring relationship can be sustained under these circumstances. There is a proliferation of services which are offered by telephone, by means of 'walk-in' centres or clinics, services which are led by nurses rather than doctors, services for a variety of specialist activities which increasingly accept self-referrals. A private clinic in the Midlands was recently advertising 'open evenings' so that busy professionals with money to spend could attend and explore the cosmetic surgery opportunities on offer on their way home from work. There are web-based dispensaries for medication which, while ostensibly available on prescription only, offer an anonymous 'online consultation' where the purchaser fills in a form which is 'reviewed by a physician'. The website will often provide a helpful list of 'prescribing indications' so that the purchaser is left in no doubt as to the symptoms he or she should fill in. There is a detectable shift in ethos towards patients being encouraged to 'take responsibility' for their health, and towards models of 'shared decision making' in the consultation itself, the emphasis of which is away from mere compliance with medical advice, towards constructs which emphasize agreement such as 'concordance'.

This is a quick smattering of vignettes representing but a few of the historical shifts in the delivery of health care. However, it should suffice to signal that we are dealing with phenomena which are rapidly changing. The result of this is that researchers seeking to understand health care consultations are constantly struggling to catch up with the developments which are taking place at the level of politics and policy and which leave their imprint on the kinds of consultations to which clients will have access.

This chapter then, in attempting to come to an understanding of health care consultations, will inevitably be out of date in detail. A literature, for example, on the delivery of diagnostic news in cancer care which addresses the role of doctors and patients has now been overtaken by events – in the UK this news is now often delivered by a nurse. However, what we hope to do is familiarize the reader with the broad trends in the study of communication processes in health care consultations. These, then, can be perhaps applied to the study of new forms of consultation as they arise in the future and can form the basis of new forms of methodology.

Getting a grip on the consultation

Despite the long history of health care consultations in one form or another, it is only relatively recently that they have been subject to sustained and systematic attempts to understand them.

Some of the more intriguing early approaches to the study of psychosocial issues in health care consultations were originated by Michael and Enid Balint in the 1950s. They had both trained as medical doctors and psychoanalysts and were keen to apply psychoanalytic insights to illuminate psychological and social processes in the consultation process and the doctor–patient relationship. Over many years the Balints ran case-discussion seminars with GPs to examine their difficulties with patients. The groups' experiences formed the basis of one of the key early contributions to the literature about consultations between doctors and patients, *The Doctor, His Patient and the Illness*. In exploring the doctor–patient relationship in depth, Balint popularized the psychoanalytic notions of transference and counter-transference among medical doctors, and was also responsible for popularizing the notion that how the doctor him- or herself is is often an important part of the treatment. Balint's premise was that initially what the patient was doing was 'proposing an illness to the doctor' (1957: 22). From the patient's initial offer of problems, the doctor decides what is allowable for discussion and may impose constraints on the range of topics to explore in the consultation on the basis of unconscious concerns. This, said Balint, was often related to something threatening in the doctor's own life. For example a doctor may not wish to explore alcoholism in a patient if they drink to excess themselves. If the patient is also reluctant to discuss the issue then this can lead to collusion and a failure to solve the underlying problem.

Discussions in a Balint group generally begin with 'has anyone a case today?' A doctor then tells a story about a patient who is bothering him or her and the group will help the doctor to identify and explore the 'blocks' which are constraining exploration and management of the patient's problem. Balint groups and methods still deliver a substantial amount of literature and retain a residual popularity among practitioners. Recently they have been identified as a means of supporting GPs traumatized by the UK's reform of the NHS (Wilke 2005) and clinical supervision and support. Even to this day, they are usually run on psychodynamic lines and often one of the group leaders is a psychotherapist.

Balint's legacy was to take psychoanalysis out of the traditional consulting room and try to popularize it with members of other caring professions. It is chiefly his legacy which is responsible for a seam of psychoanalytic thinking in theory and practice concerning the GP consultation.

Aside from early attempts to theorize and educate concerning the alleged psychodynamic aspects of the health care consultation, one of the other long running aspects to the study of interactions in health care has been to build models of the consultation process.

One of the classic typologies, originated by Byrne and Long (1976) in their volume *Doctors Talking to Patients* identifies six phases which form a logical structure to the consultation. They are generally represented as follows:

Phase I: The doctor establishes a relationship with the patient.
Phase II: The doctor either attempts to discover or actually discovers the reason for the patient's attendance.
Phase III: The doctor conducts a verbal or physical examination or both.
Phase IV: The doctor, or the doctor and the patient, or the patient (in that order of probability) consider the condition.
Phase V: The doctor and occasionally the patient detail further treatment or further investigation.
Phase VI: The consultation is terminated, usually by the doctor.

Byrne and Long were also interested in the range of verbal behaviours doctors used when talking to patients. They described a spectrum ranging from a consultation that was heavily doctor-dominated, where contributions from the patients were sidelined and excluded, to consultations that were virtually monologues by the patient, without attempts at control or direction by any input from the doctor. Between these extremes, they described a variety of intermediate styles, from closed information gathering to non-directive counselling, the use of which seemed to depend on whether the doctor was more interested in developing his or her own line of thought or the patient's.

The 1970s saw the commencement of this approach in earnest. As well as Byrne and Long (1976) there were approaches such as Stott and Davis's (1979), drawing attention to what they called '[t]he exceptional potential in each primary care consultation'. They identified four key aspects, namely:

1. Management of presenting problems
2. Modification of help-seeking behaviours
3. Management of continuing problems
4. Opportunistic health promotion.

Many of these schemes were designed with teaching in mind, as the medical schools of the developed world filled with students eager for a framework within which to learn and diligently reproduce the lists, typologies and forms of knowledge that would gain them the best marks, and educators strove for ways of assessing them objectively. We will deal with a number of related schemes in the next chapter, such as the subsequent formative models of the consultation which followed broadly similar patterns from Pendleton et al. (1984) and Neighbour (1987). For the moment let us note that the typologizing of health care encounters was often done for considerably more than reasons of scientific curiosity. There were often pedagogic motives of a most earnest kind behind the formulations which researchers and educators presented.

When we make sense of consultations in health care practice through the lens of existing literature it is important to bear in mind that this body of work is constrained in several ways.

First, it is constrained by its focus of attention. A good deal of it has been devoted to the study of doctor and patient interaction in a situation that looks a lot like a GP consultation, or a first consultation on being referred to a hospital. Of course, a great many such consultations go on and they are a worthwhile object of study in their own right, but a great deal of interactional work goes on in health care involving other people such as receptionists, cleaners, nurses, catering staff, physiotherapists, chaplains, volunteer befrienders and even between patients themselves, all of which contribute to what has been called the 'litany of the clinic'. The literature is thus still dominated by studies of doctor–patient interaction, as many scholars have noted (Candlin 2000; Candlin and Candlin 2003), despite so much health care being dispensed by professions allied to medicine. There is also a curious hierarchy in the literature inasmuch as it is studies of doctor–patient interactions which have largely found their way into mainstream social science journals. Studies of interactions between nurses and patients are still mainly ghettoized into nursing journals, despite their reliance on many of the same concepts and methodological tools as their counterparts who study doctors. This may reflect the historical priority of research on doctor–patient interaction, but may also reflect hierarchies of gender and professional prestige (Porter 2001).This focus on the part of researchers arguably reflects the kinds of hierarchies we see in health care itself, where medical dominance sets the tone of many health care activities.

Second, despite the apparently raw feel of transcriptions of interactions, complete with a variety of presentational motifs such as minutely timed pauses, phonetic spelling and esoteric punctuation that seem to guarantee their authenticity, the conversations in health care reported in the literature only present a minute trace of the great variety of interactions that take place. The modesty of this work is due in part to ethical gatekeeping. Doing any kind of research in a health care context requires that the investigator negotiate a minefield of committees governing ethics or with management or research responsibilities, as well as individual managers, practitioners and patients whose permission must be sought and informed consent gained. The increasing number of gatekeepers involved has made some researchers who once studied health care communication change tack and study other professions like the law where such constraints are as yet less restrictive. Thus we are left with a reduced field of operation, the bureaucratic background to which is often only hinted at in the research report.

Third, within the range of topics and issues covered in the research on communication between practitioners and clients a number of areas of focus dominate: general practice, cancer care, heart disease and HIV/AIDS. Yet there are other areas which are less well represented. The experience of ongoing chronic ill health where the symptoms are less well defined is under-represented despite its bread and butter status to health professionals. Again, apart from the sterling efforts of people such as Bury (2001), musculoskeletal pain is infrequently investigated. Thus, the structures of social action and linguistic practice we see represented in the literature will not necessarily translate to particular cases outside this relatively narrow range of conditions. In counselling and psychotherapy, despite the use of tape recording being pioneered in these disciplines in the 1950s by Carl Rogers and his colleagues, there has been surprisingly little fine-grained analysis of the conversations which take place, though some authors have begin advocating for it (Madill et al. 2001). Researchers, who are often also practitioners, have instead focused on describing therapeutic encounters in much broader brush strokes, as illustrating general principles relating to underlying psychic phenomena and have often been impatient with the fine grain of the conversation.

With these caveats in mind let us proceed with a consideration of consultations in health care. Like the literature itself, our account will tend to foreground consultations between doctors and patients. The exponential rise in publications on this subject in the last 20 years or so has involved researchers concentrating on issues such as the interactive achievement of diagnosis in clinical encounters (Wallston 1978; Maynard 1992; Tate 1994; Pitts 1998); compliance with recommendations (Hussey and Gilland 1989); controlling frame structures (Goffman 1974; Fisher 1991; Coupland et al. 1994); and interactional management of encounters (Coupland et al. 1994; Gill and Maynard 1995). That said, the scrutiny of interactions involving other health professionals is furnishing an increasingly large number of studies, not least concerning nurse–patient and occupational therapist–client interaction.

The picture of health: consultations in the UK

A great many visits to the doctor are made in the UK. Government sources estimated that each year, in the UK's NHS alone, there were 277 million medical and dental primary care consultations. This compares with 8.6 million hospital admissions and 24.6 million outpatient and emergency department attendances (Department of Health 2000).

The length of UK primary care consultations has increased steadily from the 1960s, and in 1998 was on average 9.36 minutes (Royal College of General Practitioners 1999; Ogden et al. 2004) rising more recently to 13.3 minutes (Royal College of General Practitioners 2004). Each full-time GP sees approximately 117 patients a week and manages 90 per cent of presenting problems without referral elsewhere. Most patients attending GP consultations present with hard-to-diagnose undifferentiated problems and the GP is under considerable time pressure in which to conduct the consultation. The combination of an ageing population and a policy of early discharge from hospitals means that GPs have to deal with more complex caseloads than they did a decade or more ago. Moreover every 10 years there is a 10 per cent increase in consultation rates being reported (Ciechanowski et al. 2002).

At the same time the intensity of knowledge and expertise needed to deal with this situation is increasing dramatically. Biomedical information is doubling every 20 years and clinicians currently need to remember over two million facts at any one time to carry out their work effectively (Wyatt 1991). This represents a fourfold increase in one physician's lifetime, and increases the likelihood of error. Indeed, medical error has come to be recognized as a leading cause of death (Sandars and Esmail 2003) with diagnostic mistakes a major contributor. Some believe that the incidence of this could be minimized by better training and wider use of protocols and diagnostic algorithms (Alberti 2001). Since 1989 there has been an exponential rise in the number of guidelines issued to GPs, but this information is fragmented and not easy to find and refer to when needed (Hibble and Pencheon 1998).

The picture we present then is not an attractive one, nor very flattering to doctors. We do not single them out because the other professions do any better; it is merely that the situation facing GPs has been spelled out in some detail. In the background literature then, consultations with GPs are depicted as numerous, brief, relating to hard-to-diagnose, undifferentiated symptoms and apt to lead to conclusions which may turn out to be mistaken in the fullness of time.

At the same time we know that these consultations are not evenly spread through the population, or even among all the patients on a GP's list. Many patients consult infrequently, but a minority of patients consult much more frequently (Bellon et al. 1999; Dowrick et al. 2000; Kapur et al. 2004). Definitions of 'frequent attendance' vary, but it is generally found that a minority of patients account for a disproportionate amount of the primary care workload. For example, Newman et al. (1999) estimated that 15 per cent of patients consume nearly two-thirds of health care costs. Gill and Sharpe (1999) concluded that those who attended consultations frequently tended to have high rates of psychiatric disorder, physical disease and social difficulties. In Kapur et al.'s (2004) study high consultation rates were associated with having negative attitudes, suffering from a higher burden of physical and psychiatric disorder, suffering health anxiety, having undergone changes in psychological distress, suffering more reported physical symptoms and demographic factors such as age and sex. That is, a typical frequent consulter was more likely to be older, female, less likely to be working full time, and to be suffering from persistent physical or mental health problems. Low consulters tended to be male, in full-time employment and have positive attitudes to their health and tended not to define themselves as having chronic conditions.

From our point of view the consultation is also intriguing because of the curious relationship between the relative powers of the people involved or 'interactants'. At the start of a consultation in general practice usually the patient is invited to set the topic, yet for the rest of the time it is very often the doctor who controls the consultation. In their book *Talk at Work* Drew and Heritage stated: 'A central theme in research on institutional interaction is that in contrast to the symmetrical relationships between speakers in ordinary conversation, institutional interactions are characteristically asymmetrical' (1992: 47).

The asymmetry of the doctor–patient relationship has been described by a number of authors (Frankel 1990, 1995; ten Have 1991: 139; Heath 1992).

Balint (1957) coined the terms doctor-centred and patient-centred. Di Caccavo et al. (2000) note that much of the research regarding medical interaction has centred around these styles of communication and their effect on patient compliance and satisfaction (Savage and Armstrong 1999). Doctors use both styles of communication (Ruusuvuori 2001), alternating between a doctor-centred approach (the doctor using his or her knowledge for the benefit of the patient) and the patient-centred style (in which the patient is seen as an expert in his or her own illness).

Occasionally, patients appear to reverse this asymmetry, sometimes by unexpectedly shifting the topic of discussion (Campion and Langdon 2004). Ten Have (1991) argues that 'asymmetry' in the consultation should always be seen as interactionally achieved, rather than as some sort of 'given'.

Barry et al. (2001) conducted a qualitative study in 35 GP practices and found that only 4 out of the 35 patients interviewed had been able to discuss with the doctor the items they had previously identified as key issues. This kind of finding has a long pedigree. In developing their model of patient-centred medicine Levenstein et al. (1986) introduced the concept of 'agendas' as the key to understanding patients. They found that doctors failed to elicit 54 per cent of patients' reasons for consulting and 45 per cent of their worries. Campion et al. (1992) showed that social and emotional agendas are the most likely issues to be under-represented in the consultation. Morris et al. (2003) detected a mismatch between the perceptions of the GP and the patient in 85 per cent of the cases they studied. In 30 per cent of the cases in their study, the GP was under the impression that the complaint in question could have been managed by the patient themselves without a visit to the surgery.

The microstructure of consultations is a topic that has intrigued a great many social researchers who have studied health care, and the interaction between doctors and patients has yielded a rich literature. Very often, to the outsider this looks esoteric, with transcriptions rendered with a variety of punctuation so as to give a sense of hesitations, overlaps, paralinguistic utterances such as 'hmm' or 'ah' and intakes of breath. Pauses are minutely timed, intonations are represented and phonetic representations of words or word fragments abound. The story of how this style of research, with its minutely transcribed details, came to be established in health care is worth retelling.

It will also provide a useful framework for understanding a good deal of what follows as this approach has provided the foundations of what we know about health care encounters.

The foundations of enquiry in health care consultations: phenomenology

Understanding the microstructure of social interaction owes a great deal to phenomenology, a movement in philosophy originating in the late nineteenth and early twentieth centuries and having a great deal of influence in the social sciences from the second half of the twentieth century onwards. Many social science sub-disciplines such as conversation analysis start from some of the same premises as phenomenology, therefore it is appropriate to spend a few moments considering what this background involves and what it has contributed to the evidence base we have concerning health care encounters.

Phenomenology originated in philosophy and aimed to undertake a systematic investigation of experience. One of the key figures in its genesis was Edmund Husserl (1859–1938), a German philosopher whose focus was upon the meanings the mind employs when it contemplates an object. Husserl introduced the term *phenomenological reduction* for his method of reflection on this dynamic ([1913]1982). Because this method concentrates on meanings that are in the mind, whether or not the object present to consciousness actually exists, Husserl said the method involves 'bracketing existence', that is, setting aside the question of the real existence of the contemplated object.

These kinds of ideas found their way into the social sciences more specifically via areas of enquiry such as 'ethnomethodology'. This originated with thinkers such as Harold Garfinkel ([1967]1984) and involves the study of everyday people's methods, focusing on the way people make sense of the world and display their understandings of it. It foregrounds the question of how people already understand the world and how they use that understanding. Ethnomethodology has often been concerned with the ways in which words are reliant for their meaning on the context in which they are used, or as Garfinkel would have it, they are 'indexical'.

A further maxim of this approach is that if you want to know about an aspect of social order then you look at the work of the people whose job it is to do it. One should seek out members of society who, in their daily lives, are responsible for the maintenance of that aspect of the social order. Sacks's (1972) original question concerned objects in public places and how it was possible to see that such objects did or did not belong to somebody. His curiosity led him to study the activities of police officers who had to decide whether cars were abandoned.

Harold Garfinkel's approach was that we should treat the 'objectivity' of social facts as an accomplishment of society's members, thus making this achievement of objectivity the focus of study. In other words people are seen to 'make' realities *in situ* as they interact. The 'bracketing of existence', recommended a century earlier in the work of Husserl, now takes the form of an agnostic stance on the part of the analyst concerning the reality the participants are describing. If we take this approach, we do not try to second guess what the 'real problem' is, that is, what the people in the encounter are trying to do. As analysts, we are not trying to do it better than them, but rather, we are attempting to discover how they do it using their conversational tools. That is, as analysts we make no assumptions as to what the problem really is. Whether in health care contexts it is a case of depression or whether the patient really does have cancer is a matter for the interactants to determine jointly. As researchers, in principle and very often in fact too, we don't know. What we can study, however, is how the members *in situ* come to know.

The study of talk as a way of constructing social realities led a number of social researchers in the late 1960s and early 1970s to the study of talk in interaction. The field of conversation analysis thus grew up around the work of Emmanuel Schegloff, Harvey Sacks and Gail Jefferson. While Harvey Sacks died tragically young, these approaches were pushed forward enthusiastically and have by now generated a large literature. Conversation analysis generally attempts to describe the orderliness, structure and sequential patterns of interaction. Sometimes this is in casual contexts and in others it is in institutional contexts such as schools, doctors' surgeries, clinics, courts and so on. Conversation analysis, or approaches inspired by it, have played a major role in the study of therapeutic encounters (Allen and Pilnick 2006).

As Drew et al. (2001) characterize it, conversation analysis focuses largely on the verbal communications which people recurrently use in interacting with one another. People are, in this view, attempting to produce meaningful action and to interpret the other's meaning. In Drew and colleagues's view, there are three key features of conversation analysis (CA):

1. Any utterances are considered to be performing social actions, such as maintaining agreement between the participants, finding out the reasons for the present situation and securing the interactant's identity as a creditable person.

2. Utterances and actions are considered to be part of sequences of action, so that what one participant says and does is occasioned by what the others have just said and done. CA thus focuses on dynamic processes of interaction from which sequences are built up.

3. These sequences appear to have stable patterns. How one participant acts and speaks can be shown to have regular, predictable consequences for how the other responds.

Social interactions are meaningful for the participants who produce them, they have a natural organization that can be discovered, and the analyst is interested in understanding the machinery, the rules and the structures that produce or constitute this orderliness. As Harvey Sacks put it there was 'order at all points'. Moreover, as far as conversation analysts are concerned that is the only order there is. From the point of view of ethnomethodology and especially conversation analysis:

> . . . the primordial site of social order is found in members' use of methodical practices to produce, make sense of and thereby render accountable, features of their local circumstances ... The socially structured character of ... any enterprise undertaken by members is thus not exterior or extrinsic to their everyday workings, but interior and intrinsic, residing in the local and particular detail of practical actions undertaken by members uniquely competent to do so.
>
> (Boden and Zimmerman 1991: 6–7)

Conversation analysis and the health care encounter

Conversation analysts try to avoid using category systems that are preformed in advance of the actual observation of the interaction, and there is a great deal of interest in the local context of the utterance or exchange. Moreover, conversation analysis has its own epistemology (theory of knowledge) in that it does not concern itself with matters that are outside the conversation. The 'bracketing of existence' is almost complete:

> No assumptions are made regarding the participants' motivations, intentions or purposes; nor about their ideas, thoughts or understandings; nor their moods, emotions or feelings, except insofar as these can demonstrably be shown to be matters that participants themselves are noticing, attending to or orienting to in the course of their interaction. Further, if and when this happens their doing so is done for all practical purposes, in and of that situated, occasioned production. What is available to the hearer for such apprehendings is similarly available to the observer.
>
> (Psathas 1995: 47)

Deploying this kind of method might seem rather restrictive, and to close down analytic possibilities. However, it has opened up a number of avenues of enquiry and has disclosed new phenomena in the *terra incognita* of clinical talk. It has also been possible to identify the sorts of functions that different techniques might perform, despite the exhortation not to look beyond the text to cognitive processes and structures which underlie the interaction. An example of this close-grained attention to actual clinical encounters yielding important new insights as to how the interactional work of health care is accomplished and is able to address policy-oriented goals and concerns can be found in Heritage and Stivers's (1999) work on medical consultations. They identified an interactional device used by doctors – the 'online commentary' – during an examination which often tends to minimize the severity of the outward signs of the illness. Phrases such as 'that's fine', 'a little bit red' or 'I don't feel any lymph node swelling' lead neatly into a decision not to prescribe in a way which carries the patient along. For example, here is an example of a doctor examining a boy who has attended with his mother for a sore throat:

```
1    Doc: Can you open your mouth for me agai:n,
2    (0.3)
3    'at's it
4    (0.7)
5    Doc: Little bit re:d (.) hm
6    (1.6) ((moving sounds))
7    Doc: Alri::ght (h)
8    ((more moving sounds))
9    .....
10   ((lines omitted))
11   .....
12   Doc: Ari:ght Michael. Can I loo:k >in your< ears
13   (0.3)
14   Mum: This o:n[e:
15   Doc: ['ank you
16   (0.9)
17   Doc: 'ats fi:ne, the other one?
```

18   (4.5)
19   Doc: ktch okha:yh
20   (0.5)
21   Doc: They're alri::ght (h). I mean there's just a li:(tt)le
22   redness in his throa:t an:d just a litt,le pinkness ther:e
23   which (.) means he's got one of tho:se co:lds that make them
24   cou:gh a lot .hh Because his chest is pe:rfectly all ri:ght
25   he ce:rtainly doesn't need (.) penicillin
26   Mum: N:o[:
27   Doc: ['r anything like tha:t .hhh hh I think the coughing ....
((continues))

(p. 1506)

With the prescription of antibiotics there has for several years in the UK been a concern that they are being over-prescribed for conditions for which they are not well suited. That is, people with viral upper respiratory tract infections may want antibiotics, yet they are generally agreed not to be effective for viral conditions. Added to this is the concern about the expense of unnecessary prescriptions and the possibility that an overly widespread use of the agents in question will lead to reduced effectiveness as the microbes develop resistance to them. From the patient's (or the patient's parents') point of view, getting the prescription may be the main reason for the consultation. Some GP practices have started using 'non-prescription' pads which explain why antibiotics are not appropriate in particular cases. In the example from Heritage and Stivers (1999) above, we can see the process of minimization in action with diminutive terms used – 'a little redness', 'a little pinkness' – so as to minimize the apparent impact of the illness and prepare the ground for the fact that a prescription will not be forthcoming at the end. The picture here is similar to that identified by Rollnick et al. (2001), where a comparable 'talking down' of symptomatology was observed. The complication introduced by Rollnick and colleagues. is that patients may not want a prescription for antibiotics quite as frequently as GPs think they do, and as a consequence it may be appropriate for practitioners to elicit from patients what their expectations are at an early stage in the consultation.

The study of the 'grain' of conversation in health care encounters can also be used to help to identify the differing approaches of professional groups. Whereas it is very often doctors whose work with patients has been studied in this way, some authors are beginning to study nurses too. An example of the way that this has been undertaken can be found in the work of Collins (2005) who provides instances of encounters between professionals and clients in diabetes care. One example to which Collins draws the reader's attention is the differences between an encounter involving a nurse and one involving a doctor, which we reproduce here:

Excerpt 1 Nurse (N) and patient (P)
1   N: So how have you been. this last year
2   you think.
3   (1.5)
4   P: phhhhhh .hh I thought (I) (1.7)

5   have done alright. =
6   N:= Right.
7   (0.7)
8   P: Until you tell me that (0.2) my
9   H([ )
10   N: [HBA1 =
11   P:= HBO1
12   (0.9)
13   N: Was a bit high.
14   (0.3)
15   P: (Was) hi:gh.
16   (0.3)
17   N: Right.
18   (0.6)
19   P: U:hm
20   (0.6)
21   N: Well you might still have (0.6) done
22   alright! (0.5) but (0.3) the fact
23   (0.8).hh that your HBA1's high.
24   (0.4) it means- (0.3) maybe s- we
25   need to (0.6) look at (0.3) (h)ow
26   you're treated really and
27   (0.6)
28   N:[[(Maybe think about) OTHer options. =
29   P: [[yeah yeah
30   [available.
31   [_yeah_.
32   (0.3)
33   N: To bring it (.) more (0.6) down to an
34   acceptable level. (0.3) so that you're
35   (0.6) fine. (0.3) you can carry on
36   be[ing =
37   P: [Yes.
38   N:= healthy and all that.
[Nurse consultation in diabetes 338–118]

(p. 788)

Excerpt 2 Doctor (D) and patient (P)
1   D: Okay I'm gunna set you target level
2   2 (0.6) er:: now that (0.5) that is:
3   um:: (0.5) results of some tests
4   (.)
5   P: Yeh
6   (.)
7   D: That we've >done from the nurse. <
8   an we we >want ah) you< (.) controlled

9   to a certain level hh (.)ˌthuh most
10   important test flthat we do is the
11   H B A 1 C
12   P: ((nods)) (0.9)
13   D: Have yuh heard of this one [before]
14   P: [y e s] =
15   = this is the: er
16   (1.3)
17   P: Erm
18   (2.0)
19   P: The actual control of the: er
20   D: Tck yeh it give [s an indication of] =
21   P: [uv (the) sugar]
22   D: = how we [ll y] our diabetes is =
23   P [(uh yeh)]
24   = con[troll]ed
25   P: [y e s]
26   (.)
27   D: It's actually ah) measuring how
28   much glucose is combined with the
29   red blood cell pigment
30   P: _(Yes)_
31   D: And because the red blood cell
32   pigment is locked up in the red
33   cells which .hh have a half life of
34   a) (.)pproximately 6 to 8 weeks.
35   .hh (.) it gives us an averaging
36   out figure over that period =
37   P: = That's right (.) yeh
38   D: .hhh now:? yours is 9 point 6
39   (0.4)
40   D: an [d that is] hi: [g h:].
41   P: [Y e s :] [that i]s high =
42   D: = Y[eh]
43   P: [Ye]h
44   D: I would like tuh see that
45   somewhere near:: (.) sih)
46   between 6 and 7 percent
[Doctor consultation in diabetes 119–338]

(p. 789)

Collins notes that several distinctions are apparent between the nurse's and the doctor's communications and their respective forms of explanation. In each excerpt, the patient is positioned differently in the construction of the assessment and accompanying explanations. In the nurse consultation, the patient is invited to contribute and presents the contrast between two possible formulations ('I thought I'd done alright, but you say I haven't'), and his interpretation helps manoeuvre the nurse's explanation into position, so that it represents a response that reconciles these apparently contrasting patient and professional viewpoints. By contrast, the doctor's explanations are not developed from the patient's talk but instead the patient's assessment follows the doctor, so he confirms rather than redresses or expands the assessment and explanations the doctor provides. In summary then, Collins argues that the nurse consultation proceeds with the patient's responsibility and behaviour while the doctor's consultation is dominated by biomedical assessments and interventions. This is reflected by the different linguistic constructions that each professional uses: the doctor deploys a more technical and specialized language, while the nurse uses language more redolent of everyday usage. She uses some of the same words the patient has employed in the surrounding talk.

In diabetes care the consultation process is the main tool used by health care professionals to monitor the client's diabetes regulation and identify any complications, provide diabetes education, attempt to motivate self-care and work with patients to make decisions about treatment (Parkin and Skinner 2003). Given that even something as apparently simple as discussing the results of a blood test can yield such different outcomes, it is clear that the implications of this need to be addressed if the current drive to place effective self-management at the heart of diabetes care is to be achieved (Department of Health 2003). At present, there is evidence that the views of clinicians and clients about the consultation are often at odds with one another (Parkin and Skinner 2003). In working with the patient to determine what decisions, goals or self-care activities are needed to enable them to deal with the issues in the management of their diabetes, Parkin and Skinner suggest that autonomy-promoting strategies should be employed which are perhaps rather akin to the kinds of interaction styles exhibited by the nurse in Collins's (2005) study. Thus, once again, the fine-grained study of conversational encounters in health care yields information of potential importance to policymakers, educators and practitioners as well as clients themselves. Moreover, from the point of view of social scientific interest we can see here traces of how broader social categories and processes are having an impact on the consultation itself. That is, the doctor and nurse roles described here can be argued to manifest the notions of gender.

Beyond the doctor–patient relationship: consultations with other health care personnel

According to a good deal of research there is a major burden of illness in the community. It is widely believed that the incidence of illness and symptoms presented by patients to health care personnel represents only the tip of the 'iceberg of illness' (Morrell 1976; Freer 1980; Scambler et al. 1981; Bentzen et al. 1989; Morris et al. 2003) with the vast bulk of illness experience remaining beneath the surface (Hannay 1979). Despite this, as Morris et al. (2003) note, GPs consider that a substantial proportion of their time is wasted by patients consulting with minor ailments. The way in which patients manage the ailments they consider to be minor has considerable implications for GP workload. If patients feel the need to consult their GP for ailments their doctor considers trivial, this may place further pressure on already overbooked appointments systems.

In response to this expanding demand for primary care appointments, increasing numbers of health care providers are exploring other avenues such as appointments with nurse practitioners, to deliver first-contact health care (Jenkins-Clark and Carr-Hill 2001; Barnes et al. 2004). Thus nurse practitioners will be engaged in patient consultations comparable to those undertaken by general practitioners. Patients may present at a primary care clinic for their health problem to be assessed by a nurse, which is then assessed and treated or referred on as appropriate.

As we have hinted in the foregoing section with an example drawn from a consultation between a diabetic patient and a specialist nurse, there has been considerable interest in the assessment and outcome of these nurse-led consultations, and in the UK they appear to be comparable to those of doctor-led consultations in terms of cost effectiveness, clinical benefits and the quality of care provided (Kinnersley et al. 2000; Venning et al. 2000; Grant et al. 2002; Horrocks et al. 2002; Marsden and Street 2004). Moreover, nurse-led primary health care consultations are generally rated as satisfactory by most patients (Poulton 1995), with high levels of satisfaction often being recorded, sometimes better than those of doctor-led consultations (Shum et al. 2000; Pritchard and Kendrick 2001; Horrocks et al. 2002).

In a study by Barratt (2005) of attendees at a nurse-led walk-in clinic, there appeared to be several different styles of interaction initiated by patients. These styles included:

- *Seekers* (patients seeking treatment) who were keen to explore all the possible avenues of treatment. For example, one patient (P9), after being told about appropriate self-care measures, said: 'Is there any other medicine I could take to help this viral infection?' (p. 334) They seemed reluctant to accept that, aside from basic self-care, there was little else that could be done and kept probing for more.
- *Clinical Presenters* (patients presenting clinical histories). For example Patient 2 (P2), opened his consultation with: 'I've had a cough for three weeks. I cough up green stuff. I've been taking cough medicines. The cough has stayed the same' (p. 335). These patients tended to appear quite happy with anything the nurse suggested, and did not appear to have preconceived ideas about appropriate courses of action. Indeed, according to the nurses they were almost too easy to please and thus gave little feedback as to whether the proffered advice was appropriate or sufficient.
- *Confirmers* (patients checking the severity of their illnesses). These tended to say things like P8: 'I think I have tonsillitis. I want to confirm that with you and see if I need to take antibiotics' (p. 335). These patients were cooperative and seemed to make the nurses feel at ease. It did not appear that they had a particular agenda, such as trying to obtain medication.
- *Seekers to Confirmers* (patients who initially seek treatment, but who change to a confirmatory style). The people in this group undertook a change in emphasis, apparently as a result of the processes ongoing in the consultation. The key feature of this group was their use of the 'voice of the lifeworld' and a

correspondent reflection of this by the nurse practitioners. The following dialogue was recorded between Patient 10 (P10) and NP 5, while awaiting the results of a throat swab test: P10: 'My job's a nightmare. I've been overdoing it, burning the candle at both ends'. NP5: 'Maybe your immune system is run down, have you had any days off work? You need to be careful and look after yourself'. P10: [not recorded verbatim] says that he has been working a lot. NP5: 'Yes, this is negative [throat swab result], so there's no bacteria, I think you need to get some rest. This could be stress. You need to recharge your batteries. I don't think you need antibiotics. There is nothing to treat with antibiotics'. P10: 'I don't want to take antibiotics for the sake of antibiotics' (p. 336). In this example, once these lifeworld issues had been introduced by the patient and the nurse had responded, the consultation agenda shifted from one of seeking to a more confirmatory orientation of checking the severity of their illnesses and accepting self-care health advice.

- *Anticipators* (patients who anticipate their need for treatment). The Antici-pators typically presented a history which described their prior experience of the current illness they thought they had. Patient 14 exemplifies this concise history style: 'I think I've got tonsillitis. Basically, I've got a very swollen throat. I've had it before' (p. 337).

The nurses acknowledged this anticipatory self-presentation style and responded with clinically focused history taking. This continued as the consultation progressed, and resulted in clinically led advice concerning the correct use of the antibiotics they were given.

In Barratt's study, the nurse practitioners flexibly modified their communication strategies in response to the patients' self-presentation styles. In Barratt's view, this helped to resolve any tensions between the patients' expressed reasons for coming in for a consultation, and their needs for treatment as reflected in the nurses' clinical assessments.

In these examples there is a common theme of cooperation underlying the consultations. That is, the client and the health professional are jointly embarked on a journey to discover the seat of the problem, to determine a course of action or a suitable treatment. There may be some divergence of expectations concerning the severity of the problem or whether medication is necessary, but to a large extent we can take for granted a consensus between the interactants concerning the nature of the consultation.

Conclusion: extending the picture

As we have described, the impetus from phenomenology, ethnomethodology and conversation analysis has yielded a number of studies seeking to explore the micro-structure of the conversation, some of which have yielded new phenomena to analysts and practitioners. Once they have been identified they often yield an 'aha! experience' on the part of the reader who can perhaps recall similar structures of social action on his or her own encounters with practitioners. This then provides a powerful and persuasive means for characterizing what health communication is about and how the actors or interactants accomplish it. In the mundane details of describing a pain, looking at the physical signs, or discussing the symptoms there are some of the most exquisitely detailed conversational works in progress. Yet at the same time, to characterize the 'picture of health' we might do well to look at other things too. The broader matrix of people's lives has often been rather difficult to connect to the clinical encounter. The often complex, morally ambiguous and frequently frightening progress of illness which we touched upon in the chapter about narratives is one way of getting a grip on this. Equally, the exploration of people's lives and community experiences is currently less the territory of the scholar of communication and more the kind of thing that is dealt with by the essayist, the storyteller or the film-maker.

Greenhalgh and Hurwitz (1998) highlight the gap that often exists between patients' and doctors' narratives about health and illness. Health care professionals', especially doctors', narratives tend to centre upon disease and its cure through the application of scientific medicine. On the other hand lay people may see things differently. For them, health may be seen as independent of disease and illness and, as Radley (1994) notes, has meaning in terms of feelings and capacities involving one's ability to participate in physical and social activities. Psychological and epidemiological research indicates that social support and social power make a substantial contribution to health (Kernick et al. 1999). Perhaps, as Kernick et al. (1999) suggest, patients may be seeking support and empowerment through medical consultations more than their doctors realize, and perhaps also nurses place a higher value than do doctors on the 'caring' perspective which involves responsiveness to patients' wishes.

So the larger scale meaning of encounters in people's lives is sometimes difficult to relate to the microstructures of clinical encounters at the present state of knowledge. Equally, there are other aspects of the microstructure of conversation of which we know far less. Sometimes the most interesting aspects of interaction take place outside formal consultations. What is missing from the body of literature about the microstructure of these accounts is any sense of the communication that goes on in corridors, common rooms or out in the 'community'. As we shall argue later, researchers might usefully adopt a focus on events which might occur naturalistically outside the consulting room, but which might turn out to be rich with the same kind of detailed microarchitecture as the consultations which have been studied by conversation analysts. Later, we will consider how one might begin to study this 'wildtrack' communication, and the contribution this might make to caring or healing work.

References

Alberti, K.G. (2001) Medical errors: a common problem, *British Medical Journal*, 322: 501–2.

Allen, D. and Pilnick, A. (eds) (2006) *The Social Organization of Healthcare Work*. Oxford: Blackwell.

Balint, M. (1957) *The Doctor, His Patient and the Illness*. New York: International Universities Press.

Barnes, H., Crumbie, A., Carlisle, C. and Pilling, D. (2004) Patients' perceptions of 'uncertainty' in nurse practitioner consultations, *British Journal of Nursing*, 13: 1350–4.

Barratt, J. (2005) A case study of styles of patient self-presentation in the nurse practitioner primary health care consultation, *Primary Health Care Research and Development*, 6: 329–40.

Barry, C., Stevenson, F.A, Britten, N., Barber, N. and Bradley. C. (2001) Giving voice to the lifeworld: more humane, more effective medical care? A qualitative study of doctor–patient communication in general practice, *Social Science and Medicine*, 53: 487–505.

Bellon, J.A., Delgado, A., Luna, J.D. and Lardelli, P. (1999) Psychosocial and health belief variables associated with frequent attendance in primary care, *Psychological Medicine*, 29: 1347–57.

Bentzen, N., Christiansen, T. and Pedersen, K.M. (1989) Self-care within a model for demand for medical care, *Social Science and Medicine*, 29: 185–93.

Boden, D. and Zimmerman, D.H. (1991) *Talk and Social Structure: Studies in Ethnomethodology and Conversation Analysis*. Cambridge: Polity Press.

Bury, M. (2001) Illness narratives: fact or fiction? *Sociology of Health and Illness*, 23: 263–85.

Byrne, P.S. and Long, B.E.L (1976) *Doctors Talking to Patients*. London: HMSO.

Campion, P.D. and Langdon, M. (2004) Achieving multiple topic shifts in primary care medical consultations: a conversation analysis study in UK general practice, *Sociology of Health and Illness*, 261: 81–101.

Campion, P.D., Butler, N.M. and Cox, A.D. (1992) Principle agendas of doctors and patients in general practice consultations, *Family Practitioner*, 9: 181–90.

Candlin, C.N. and Candlin, S. (2003) Health care communication: A problematic site for applied linguistics research, *Annual Review of Applied Linguistics*, 23: 134–54.

Candlin, S. (2000) New dynamics in the nurse–patient relationship?, in S. Sarangi and M. Coulthard (eds) *Discourse and Social Life*. London: Longman.

Ciechanowski, P.S., Hirsch, I.B. and Katon, W.J. (2002) Interpersonal predictors of HbA(1c) in patients with type 1 diabetes, *Diabetes Care*, 25: 731–6.

Collins, S. (2005) Explanations in consultations: the combined effectiveness of doctors' and nurses' communication with patients, *Medical Education*, 39: 785–96.

Coupland, J., Robinson, J.D. and Coupland, N. (1994) Frame negotiation in doctor–elderly patient interactions, *Discourse and Society*, 5: 89–124.

Department of Health (2000) *The NHS Plan*. London: Department of Health.

Department of Health (2003) *The National Framework for Diabetes: Standards*. London: Department of Health.

Di Caccavo, A., Ley, A. and Reid, F. (2000) What do practitioners discuss with their patients? Exploring the relationship between content and medical consultations and treatment decisions, *Journal of Health Psychology*, 5(1): 87–98.

Dowrick, C.F., Bellon, J.A. and Gomez, M.J. (2000) GP frequent attendance in Liverpool and Granada: the impact of depressive symptoms, *British Journal of General Practice*, 50: 361–5.

Drew, P. and Heritage, J. (eds) (1992) *Talk at Work: Interaction in Institutional Settings*. Cambridge: Cambridge University Press.

Drew, P., Chatwin, J. and Collins, S. (2001) Conversation analysis: A method for research into interactions between patients and health care professionals, *Health Expectations*, 4: 58–70.

Fisher, S. (1991) A discourse of the social: Medical talk/power talk/oppositional talk, *Discourse and Society*, 2: 157–82.

Frankel, R.M. (1990) Talking in interviews: a dispreference for patient-initiated questions in physician–patient encounters, in G. Psathas (ed.) *Interaction Competence*. Washington, DC: University Press of America.

Frankel, R.M. (1995) Some answers about questions in clinical interviews, in G.H. Morris and R.J. Chenail (eds) *The Talk of the Clinic: Explorations in the Analysis of Medical and Therapeutic Discourse*. Hillsdale, NJ: Lawrence Erlbaum Associates.

Freer, C.B. (1980) Self-care: a health diary study, *Medical Care*, 18: 853–61.

Garfinkel, H. ([1967]1984) *Studies in Ethnomethodology*. Cambridge: Polity Press.

Gill, D. and Sharpe, M. (1999). Frequent consulters in general practice: a systematic review of studies of prevalence, associations and outcome, *Journal of Psychosomatic Research*, 47: 115–30.

Gill, V.T. and Maynard, D.W. (1995) On labelling in actual interaction: delivering and receiving diagnoses of developmental disabilities, *Social Problems*, 42(1): 11–37.

Goffman, E. (1974) *Frame Analysis*. New York: Harper and Row.

Grant, C., Nicholas, R., Moore, L. and Salisbury, C. (2002) An observational study comparing quality of care in walk-in centres with general practice and NHS Direct using standardized patients, *British Medical Journal*, 324, 1556–9.

Greenhalgh, T. and Hurwitz, B. (1998) *Narrative Based Medicine*. London: BMJ Books.

Hannay, D.R. (1979) *The Symptom Iceberg: A Study of Community Health*. London: Routledge and Kegan Paul.

Heath, C. (1992) Diagnosis in the general practice consultation, in P. Drew and J. Heritage (eds) *Talk at Work: Interaction in Institutional Settings*. Cambridge: Cambridge University Press.

Heritage, J. and Stivers, T. (1999) Online commentary in acute medical visits: a method of shaping patient expectations, *Social Science and Medicine*, 49: 1501–17.

Hibble, A. and Pencheon, D. (1998) Guidelines in general practice: the new Tower of Babel? *British Medical Journal*, 317: 862–33.

Horrocks, S., Anderson, E. and Salisbury, C. (2002) Systematic review of whether nurse practitioners working in primary care can provide equivalent care to doctors, *British Medical Journal*, 324: 819–23.

Husserl, E. ([1913]1982) *Ideas Pertaining to a Pure Phenomenology and to a Phenomenological Philosophy – First Book: General Introduction to a Pure Phenomenology* (translated by F. Kersten). The Hague: Martinus Nijhoff.

Hussey, L.C. and Gilland, K. (1989) Compliance, low literacy and locus of control, *Nursing Clinics of North America*, 24(3): 605–11.

Jenkins-Clarke, S. and Carr-Hill, R. (2001) Changes, challenges and choices for the primary health care workforce: looking to the future, *Journal of Advanced Nursing*, 34: 842–49.

Kapur, N., Hunt, I., Lunt, M., McBeth, J., Creed, F. and MacFarlane, G. (2004) Psychosocial and illness related predictors of consultation rates in primary care – a cohort study, *Psychological Medicine*, 34: 719–28.

Kernick, D.P., Reinhold, D.M. and Mitchell, A. (1999) How should patients consult? A study of the differences in viewpoint between doctors and patients, *Family Practice*, 16: 562–5.

Kinnersley, P., Anderson, E., Parry, K. et al. (2000) Randomized controlled trial of nurse practitioner versus general practitioner care for patients requesting 'same day' consultations in primary care, *British Medical Journal*, 320: 1043–8.

Levenstein, J.H., McCracken, E.C., McWhinney, I.R., Stewart, M. and Brown, J.B. (1986) The patient-centred clinical method 1: a model for the doctor–patient interaction in family medicine, *Family Practice*, 3: 24–30.

Lynch, M. (1993) *Scientific Practice and Ordinary Action: Ethnomethodological and Social Studies of Science*. Cambridge: Cambridge University Press.

Madill, A., Widdicombe, S. and Barkham, M. (2001) The potential of conversation analysis for psychotherapy research, *Counselling Psychologist*, 29(3): 413–34.

Marsden, J. and Street, C. (2004) A primary health care team's views of the nurse practitioner role in primary care, *Primary Health Care Research and Development*, 5: 17–27.

Maynard, D.W. (1992) On clinicians co-implicating recipients' perspective in the delivery of diagnostic news, in P. Drew and J. Heritage (eds) *Talk at Work: Interaction in Institutional Settings*. Cambridge: Cambridge University Press.

Morrell, D.C. (1976) Symptoms perceived and recorded by patients, *Journal of the Royal College of General Practitioners*, 26: 398–403.

Morris, C.J., Cantrill, J.A. and Weiss, M.C. (2003) Minor ailment consultations: a mismatch of perceptions between patients and GPs, *Primary Health Care Research and Development*, 4: 365–70.

Neighbour, R. (1987) *The Inner Consultation: How to Develop an Effective and Intuitive Consulting Style*. Lancaster: MTP Press.

Newman, E., Walker, E. and Gefland, A. (1999) Assessing the ethical costs and benefits of trauma focused research, *General Hospital Psychiatry*, 21: 187–96.

Ogden, J., Bavalia, K., Bull, M. et al. (2004) 'I want more time with my doctor': a quantitative study of time and the consultation, *Family Practice*, 21(5): 479–83.

Parkin, T. and Skinner, T.C. (2003) Discrepancies between patient and professionals' recall and perception of an outpatient consultation, *Diabetic Medicine*, 20: 909–14.

Pendleton, D., Havelock, P., Schofield, T. and Tate, P. (1984) *The Consultation, Learning and Teaching*. Oxford: Oxford University Press.

Pitts, M. (1998) The medical consultation, in M. Pitts and K. Phillips (eds) *The Psychology of Health*. London: Routledge.

Porter, S. (2001) Women in a women's job: the gendered experience of nurses, in W.C. Cockerham and M.L. Glasser (eds) *Readings in Medical Sociology*. Englewood Cliffs, NJ: Prentice Hall.

Poulton, B. (1995) Keeping the customer satisfied, *Primary Health Care*, 5: 16–19.

Pritchard, A. and Kendrick, D. (2001) Practice nurse and health visitor management of acute minor illness in a general practice, *Journal of Advanced Nursing*, 36: 556–62.

Psathas, G. (1995) *Conversation Analysis: The Study of Talk in Interaction*. London: Sage.

Radley, A. (1994) *Making Sense of Illness*. London: Sage.

Rollnick, S., Seale, C., Rees, M., Butler, C., Kinnersley, P. and Anderson, L. (2001) Inside the routine general practice consultation: an observational study of consultations for sore throats, *Family Practice*, 18: 506–10.

Royal College of General Practitioners (1999) *General Practice Workload*. Information sheet No 3. London: Royal College of General Practitioners.

Royal College of General Practitioners (2004) *RCGP Information Sheet No.3: General Practitioner Workload* (April). London: Royal College of General Practitioners.

Ruusuvuori, J. (2001) Looking means listening: coordinating displays of engagement in doctor–patient interaction, *Social Science and Medicine*, 52: 1093–108.

Sacks, H. (1972) Notes on police assessment of moral character, in D. Sudnow (ed.) *Studies in Social Interaction*. Glencoe: Free Press.

Sandars, J. and Esmail, A. (2003) The frequency and nature of medical error in primary care: understanding the diversity across studies, *Family Practice*, 20(3): 231–6.

Savage, R. and Armstrong, D. (1999) Effect of a general practitioner's consulting style on patient satisfaction: a controlled study, *British Medical Journal*, 301: 968–70.

Scambler, A., Scambler, G. and Craig, D. (1981) Kinship and friendship networks and women's demand for primary care, *Journal of the Royal College of General Practitioners*, 31: 746–50.

Shum, C., Humphreys, A., Wheeler, D., Cochrane, M., Skoda, S. and Clement, S. (2000) Nurse management of patients with minor illnesses in general practice: multicentre, randomized controlled trial, *British Medical Journal*, 320: 1038–43.

Stott, N.C.H. and Davis, R.H. (1979) The exceptional potential in each primary care consultation, *Journal of the Royal College of General Practitioners*, 29: 201–5.

Tate, P. (1994) *The Doctor's Communication Handbook*. Oxford: Radcliffe Medical Press.

ten Have, P. (1991) Talk and institution: a reconsideration of the 'asymmetry' of doctor–patient interaction, in D. Boden and D. Zimmerman (eds) *Talk and Social Structure*. Cambridge: Polity Press.

Venning, P., Durries, A., Roland, M., Roberts, C. and Lease, B. (2000) Randomized controlled trial comparing cost effectiveness of general practitioners and nurse practitioners in primary care, *British Medical Journal*, 320: 1048–53.

Wallston, T.S. (1978) *Three Biases in the Processing of Diagnostic Information*. Chapel Hill, NC: Psychometric Laboratory, University of North Carolina.

Wilke, G. (2005) Beyond Balint: a group-analytic support model for traumatized doctors, *Group Analysis*, 38(2): 265–80.

Wyatt, J.C. (1991) Use and sources of medical knowledge, *Lancet*, 338: 1368–73.

6 Teaching communication traditionally: chalk, talk and role plays

Histories of advice

Over the last several millennia there has been a great deal of advice dispensed as to how physicians – and presumably other health professionals – should conduct themselves. Much of this prefigures the kinds of advice and education which are provided to trainee practitioners today.

In the European Renaissance, Francois Rabelais (1494–1553) advised that when doctors present themselves to their patients they should be well dressed, with beards trimmed and hands and finger nails clean. But, above all else, they should be cheerful and serene because a gloomy doctor makes a patient fear a poor prognosis and may even help to cause it, whereas cheerful and serene humours communicate themselves to the sufferer (MacLean 1994: 803).

This Renaissance revolution of which Rabelais was a part has its echoes in the present time. The last half century has famously seen a revolution in the kinds of communication which are encouraged between clients and health care providers. Since Hildegard Peplau (1952) famously drew attention to the role of interpersonal processes in nursing just over half a century ago there has been a massive investment in research and training in communication skills for student health professionals.

A great many approaches to communication skills developed over the last half century have been informed by the discourse of counselling (Bowles et al. 2001). The legacy of nondirective 'rogation' counselling techniques does not necessarily leave the practitioner with a system that has very much utility at the bedside, but this approach still forms the backbone of many communication skills programmes (Bowles et al. 2001: 347). Indeed, so pervasive is the influence of counselling models that Suikkala and Leino-Kilpi (2001) use the terms 'nursing' and 'counselling' interchangeably as does Nagano (2001: 25), who states that 'the demands of nursing require the nurse to play counselor with the patient' and argues that the object of nursing communication is to enter the client's private world. Suikkala and Leino-Kilpi (2001: 48) discuss 'empathetic ability', the 'development of counseling skills' and 'active listening' in a person-centred relationship as being somehow fundamental to good health care. These kinds of approaches are becoming increasingly modish in other health care disciplines too, such as health visiting and occupational therapy. Also, in social care disciplines the pervasiveness of these ideas can be noted. In a sense, the therapeutic encounter or the consultation itself are increasingly seen as part of the therapy.

As Bowles et al. (2001) note, these kinds of perspectives which have proliferated in the past few decades are often based on the assumption that one can form a nondirective relationship – of the kind that exists in counselling situations – with a client over a long period of time. Of course, in practical settings, few nurses have the time or opportunity to fulfil this function, even if patients were to demand it, which they may not. Furthermore, others claim that there is no robust evidence to say that counselling is effective in secondary medical or acute areas (Bowles et al. 2001).

This chapter will therefore look at the question of skills and education in two complementary ways. First, we shall look at the politics of skill. That is, we will try to show how the contemporary focus on skills in the health care workforce is part of a number of broader economic, cultural and political trends in the globalized economy. Developing skills is about far more than practising a set of techniques and tells us something about how the world works, how the people in it are created, the qualities they are supposed to exhibit, the demeanour they affect, the questions they ask and the mindset to which they subscribe, all of which can be seen as connected to larger scale developments in the way that cultures and economies function. This much then is by way of background. The second part of the chapter will consider what is in the foreground, by way of training, education and learning. We will review some of the popular frameworks for making sense of the health care encounter that have been used by practitioners, educators and students. There have been many attempts to teach and examine clinical skills by means of role-playing exercises, and a number of accounts of clinical encounters in the form of structured lists, typologies and frameworks. These function not to provide a literal description of what goes on in clinical encounters but to create a framework within which learning might take place. Finally, we will suggest how there might be other possibilities for the pedagogies involved in the creation of a new generation of inventive, flexible, and communication-competent clinical practitioners for the health care world of the twenty-first-century.

The new practitioner: the politics, economics and ethics of creating practitioners

The nature of training for health care practitioners is intimately bound up with a society's ideas about the kind of practitioner it wants to create, or, in the case of continuing professional development, the kind of practitioner existing health professionals want to turn themselves into. The question also connects to more global issues relating to the nature of health care labour markets in late modernity, where health care industries are coming to constitute increasingly large proportions of the economies of many developed nations. Moreover, with the globalization of markets in health care it may well be that a practitioner trains in one country, works in another and retires to a different one to become a consumer of health care services him- or herself. Eastwood et al. (2005) describe the global migration of health care workers, especially doctors, out of regions such as sub-Saharan Africa and into the UK. Patients may be taken to their local accident and emergency unit if they collapse in the street, but for some elective and non-emergency procedures they may look abroad for treatment in increasing numbers, leading to the phenomenon of global 'health tourism'.

In the light of this, the question of what constitutes a good practitioner of health care is not easily answered. It is relatively easy to suggest that a bad practitioner is one who practises badly and who fails, for example, to exhibit specific competencies in caring for patients. However, the opposite does not seem to be entirely true, as Duncan et al. (2003) note. The practitioners who labour through all the advice in guides to 'good practice' – even if they do so consistently and over a long period of time – are not necessarily 'good practitioners'; even if the most diligent of examiners ticks all the boxes on the evaluation sheet. They may be technically competent in following the rules, but they may still not seem to have the right kind of disposition towards their patients or clients. The nature of this disposition, say Duncan and colleagues, may be that of 'caring'. In a sense, does the practitioner care? However, as Gorovitz (1994) has argued, the vague and ephemeral nature of this concept poses substantial difficulties. It would, after all, be very difficult to rate this in medical or nursing students.

In nursing itself, there has often been a tension between the kinds of skills that different groups would like to see the nurse display. Equally, there has always been concern that education is not necessarily good for nursing. As recently as 1970 Young put it thus: 'The aim of nursing education should be to produce a good nurse, not necessarily a *well educated* young woman' (1970: 174). This in turn echoes Florence Nightingale's sentiments over a century earlier that to be a good nurse was to be a good woman. Nightingale was working at a time when nursing was being dragged away from the popular image of drunken 'Mrs. Gamp' midwives towards notions of moral propriety more attuned to middle-class Victorian tastes. More recently still, an editorial leader in *The Observer* (2006) deemed nursing a 'practical' subject, like catering, which has become 'cluttered ... with spurious academic theory'. So even today, some people consider it to be little more than perhaps an activity as 'practical' and obvious as sticking a pie in the oven.

Thus, the values that inform our choices about what skills, attributes and dispositions to develop in trainee practitioners reflect more widely held social values, norms and assumptions about what it means to be, say, a doctor, nurse, paramedic or physiotherapist. There is nowadays a more or less universal recognition that communication skills are a key element of any contemporary clinician's skill repertoire and are essential to their competence (Kurtz et al. 1998). As we have seen so far, there is also widespread agreement that patient-centred communication, using open questions, and trying to elicit the patient's full range of concerns and problems improves patients' health status and increases the efficiency of care by reducing the need for supplementary diagnostic tests and referrals (Stewart et al. 2000; Chan et al. 2003). The emphasis on the need for communication skills training is echoed in the literature on nursing skills over the last 20 years (Wilkinson et al. 1999; Bowles et al. 2001; Suikkala and Leino-Kilpi 2001).

Despite many such initiatives, however, there have been some concerns that practitioners are not learning the set of skills that are alleged to underlie good communication in a way which improves daily practice. There is some evidence that training does not significantly enhance practice in clinical areas (Booth et al. 1999; Wilkinson et al. 1999). Bowles et al. (2001) suggest that this finding may be accounted for by a lack of role models or clinically credible educators. Equally, they say, it may be because the education and training make use of concepts derived from counselling that are difficult to implement in clinical practice.

A further problem with much communication skills training was identified nearly 30 years ago when Fielding and Llewelyn (1979) complained that many communications skills training programmes in nursing did not provide a theoretical framework that was applicable to all nursing's fields of endeavour. This view has been taken up periodically over the intervening period by those who argue that current approaches to communication skills training are inadequate and that training should provide a greater range of skills within a coherent theoretical framework (Crute et al. 1989; Bowles et al. 2001). Thus, despite the already heavy investment in training in 'skills', it is argued that if only the educators did more of it, or were better role models, or appeared to have a consistent theoretical framework, or were more effective communicators themselves, or had more of this or less of that, training would work better. Now of course many of these accounts are written by people whose careers are based in teaching student practitioners their communication skills, so it is not surprising that they advocate a greater role for themselves and their colleagues in the curriculum, nor should it be surprising that they advocate that their particular theoretical framework should supervene over the allegedly stultifying influence of biomedicine. However, as we shall suggest in the next section, maybe the problem is more fundamental than that. It may not be so easily amenable to solution through enhancements in 'training' or 'skills'.

'Skills' and the discourses of education

In order to place the contemporary fascination with the acquisition of communication and consultation skills in context we would first like to take the reader on a short detour into social theory. We will deal with some of the frameworks and techniques for teaching a little later, but first we would like to ask where this fascination with communication skills has come from. Many of the great feats of human civilization have taken place without anyone being trained in 'communication skills' at all.

The growing interest in communication skills in the training of health care professionals has gone hand in hand with a number of other trends in the education system. Legislation and policy from successive governments have attempted to gear education more closely to the occupational marketplace. Throughout the contemporary education system in the UK there is a view – evident for instance in the Dearing Report of the late 1990s entitled *Higher Education in the Learning Society* (Dearing 1997) – that education is a vocationally oriented transmission of knowledge and skills. What is perhaps most distinctive about this view of education is its focus upon the teaching, learning and practising of 'key skills'. These are seen as valuable occupationally and are believed to be transferable from one sphere of life to another, from the classroom to the workplace, for example. Moreover, they are seen to be the basis for future success in a person's profession, and successful 'lifelong learning'. The discourses of 'skills' and the political climate in which they flourish require careful scrutiny because the terms carry 'unspoken assumptions and connotations that can powerfully influence the discourses they permeate – in part by constituting a body of *doxa*, or taken-for-granted commonsense belief that escapes critical scrutiny' (Fraser 1997: 121).

As Butterwick and Benjamin (2006) suggest, it is as if future professionals – or indeed future citizens as a whole – are being asked to invest in themselves by acquiring 'skills'. At the same time, however, new forms of subtle institutionalization and standardization are taking place to ensure that the newly trained workers have the specific professional skills to do their jobs. But as Butterwick and Benjamin note, there is more to the current definition of skills than this – 'skills' now include the right attitudes and dispositions, especially a willingness to be adaptable and flexible: 'Success will come to those who know themselves – their strengths and values, how they best perform, where they belong and what they should contribute' (Opengart and Short 2002: 222).

We should note that the term 'skills' in this sense does not necessarily mean that the clients of these practitioners will feel any better. The discourse of 'skills' in contemporary educational life is not necessarily attached to any manifest proficiency in the practice of making people feel better, but rather refers to a way of conceptualizing the learning process and the learner him- or herself (Contu et al. 2003).

In addition, something intriguing has happened to the way we see communication processes over the last half century. Whereas once these kinds of activities were presumed to be cultivated informally and medical or nursing education was about attending to physical aspects of care – anatomy, biochemistry, blanket baths and the like – nowadays communication is one of those areas which has become increasingly professionalized. As Furedi (2004) remarks, areas of life which were once dominated by communitarian ties, comfortable assumptions concerning shared meanings and informal practices are increasingly subject to professional trainings. Indeed, as Furedi argues, the individual management of communication and feeling is less favoured in contemporary culture. Preference is given instead to collective projects of training in the acquisition of skills as a way of adding value to oneself as a practitioner. Training in communication skills then can be seen as part of a broader project of professionalization. The individual has added value to themselves by participating in these collective exercises of training in 'skills'.

Seeing communicative processes in health care as a set of skills that can be learned through communally undertaken instruction and practice has its drawbacks. Let us focus on three kinds of problems here. First, in order to make this out to be a worthwhile activity, we must assume that a communication skill, once learnt, can be readily transferred from one context to another. Yet when we look at the specific manifestations of even the most widely dispersed communicative practice, says Fairclough (2003), it is always locally recontextualized, transformed and appropriated. In the case of health care it is dubious whether a set of communication and consultation skills built upon a counselling model, where it is assumed that the client and practitioner have a 50-minute hour in which to conduct their business, will be appropriate to a momentary communication event in the corridor of a busy hospital, or in a 10-minute consultation with a GP.

Second, seeing therapeutic interventions and health care events in terms of skills involves assuming that there is a simple relationship between what a person actually says or does by way of social practice, and the 'skills' in question. It is as if the internalized models of what to say and how to act are primary and that the discourse is merely an instantiation of the underlying model (Fairclough 1989). As Nelson-Jones

(2002: 118) quotes approvingly: 'One of the Buddha's sayings is: "As the shadow follows the body, as we think, so we become." Put another way, skilful communication and action follows from skilful thinking'. As the reader might anticipate, this seems to us to imply an overly simplistic model of communicative processes between human beings, and seems to imply a curious nominalism, such that cognition is seen as a precedent of action. Language as it is spoken in rich and variegated contexts involves a complex matching of models with immediate needs. The emergent communications may be radically different from any model, involve a partial resemblance to a model or display a baffling mixture of models. Creativity or collective practice may have more impact than skill *per se*.

Thirdly, and most seriously, it is assumed that there is a given and accepted way of using language to do certain things, as if discourse was a simple and relatively universal matter of technique. However, as critical theorists such as Fairclough (2003) remind us, in many forms of life the way in which language gets to be used has often come about as a result of the operation of power. One way of speaking comes about through excluding, marginalizing and opposing other ways. As we saw in the first chapter, some kinds of language and culture may be endowed with more cultural capital than others, may be ascribed to a social habitus of greater value, or may be closer to the speech of those who set the rules of the game in any given social situation. Equally, ways of using language within any social practice are socially contestable. From this point of view, a reduction of communication in therapeutic settings to a set of 'skills', in Fairclough's view, would enable powerful individuals to impose the sort of social practices they favour, by getting people to see them as mere techniques.

All too often, students and educators come to regard communication skills as an unengaging chore, without reliable means to ensure good performance. Yet if the laudable but often rather vague aims of central policy initiatives are to be achieved, health care professionals need to work with service users in ways that facilitate health benefits. Many health professionals work in a positive way, often in stressful and under-resourced contexts, to achieve this (Hart et al. 2001).

Despite all the emphasis that has been placed on communication skills and the extent to which the whole business of communication has come within the purview of professionalism in health care, there are still many accounts, especially from service users, of how interactions between them and health and social care professionals and institutions result in their feeling oppressed and humiliated, rather than cared for (Bloor and McIntosh 1990; Edwards and Popay 1994; Hart et al. 2001).

From the point of view of service users, the situation may look very bleak indeed. Ill health is associated with economic disadvantage and social exclusion, so some of those who need services the most acutely may be most disadvantaged. It may, say Hart et al. (2001) result in inequalities in access to care being exacerbated. In the case of doctors, some have expressed concerns that training actually makes practitioners worse: 'It is difficult to equate the delightful, caring, and extremely gifted young people who one encounters on their entry to medical school with some of the horror stories ... of disturbingly callous and rude behaviour' (Weatherall 1994: 527). There are many complex debates behind these issues, implicating 'resourcing issues', organizational politics and culture. The history of education and training in the health care professions over the last hundred years is littered with personal accounts of people who have felt that they have somehow changed for the worse as a result of their training; that organizational and institutional factors have defeated their humanitarian impulses.

Modern sensibilities have added accounts of oppression and inequality based around class, gender, disability, sexuality, ethnicity and socio-economic status to the panoply of reasons why students may not fare well in training and education regimes and why patients may not fare well at the hands of people who have been trained in this way. Ensuring that health care professionals can work with disadvantaged clients so as to sensitively take account of differences in background, values and lifestyle, and to respect human rights and promote human dignity is of major importance in achieving policy objectives which set the patient at the heart of care.

Clearly, no matter how we try to train the rising generation of health professionals this will not be an easy task. It challenges and burdens a body of people who are often under a great deal of stress themselves already, and who are members of professions already facing problems retaining the staff they currently have. The literature on stress in the health and social professions is testament to this (Newton et al. 1996; Weinberg and Creed 2000).

Thus, the task of acquiring the skills necessary to communicate with clients involves a number of conceptually fraught and politically contentious processes. The very fact that we talk about skills at all in the context of communication is open to debate – the activities involved do not necessarily cleave neatly into trainable and testable transferable skills; this understanding of the world itself reflects the economics and politics of the education and health care systems. We also have the task, if we are educators or practitioners, of acquiring and transmitting the desiderata of good communication in institutional circumstances that tend to make it difficult. What McCue (1982) wrote about trainee doctors in paediatrics over 20 years ago could just as easily be true today: 'Among four paediatric intern groups, residents had more negative attitudes towards patients, worsened physician–patient relationships, and decreased positivity about life at the end of the internship year compared with the beginning' (p. 458). Contact with actual patients during clinical work (the 'internship year') made matters worse, in other words.

Thus, we have an apparently paradoxical situation. On the one hand, people may gain in experience in the health care professions but this growing expertise and experience can be accompanied by the impoverishment of their actual practice and a more negative outlook on patients. As Robinson et al. (2003) point out, experience and expertise constitute a conundrum. On the one hand, they are great assets to the practitioner. Indeed, in Kant's view experience is all that any of us can have. Yet 'experience' may also make us progressively more resistant to change. Equally, experience is a valuable resource in teaching. Many educators take the view that teaching is most effective when it includes recognition of learner's previous experience (Robinson et al. 2003).

Giving practitioners measurable skills: the objective structured clinical examination

This fourth section represents the transition between the first part of the chapter where we dealt with the culture, politics, and economics of the health care environment. Now, let us examine some of the practices, frameworks and theories that can be found in the education of future health care professionals. Let us begin with one of the curiosities facing any observer of the training process in health care communication. That is, the ubiquity of role playing in the curriculum or the assessment process. The use of these kinds of simulations, plus the closely related assessment technique, the 'OSCE' (objective structured clinical examination) which often uses role-played events on which students are graded, has gained near universal acceptance in education for health professionals since it was developed in 1975 as a means of clinical competence assessment (Harden et al. 1975). Many professional trainings involve OSCEs to assess students' interactional skills and to ensure that they include all the elements which are deemed necessary in a clinical encounter. Despite their relatively recent origins – within the living memory of some practitioners – their present-day popularity is one of the great success stories of contemporary education for clinicians.

In the teaching and learning arena, OSCEs have grown to have an important role in the clinical learning process by providing exposure of medical students to standardized patients or real patients in various clinically relevant situations designed by medical or nursing school faculties. Auewarkarul et al. (2005) describe using a comprehensive battery of assessment using OSCE 'stations' to examine history taking and diagnoses, as well as procedural skills and even laboratory activities, though in the UK they are more usually confined to the clinical skills used at the bedside or the consulting room.

The reliability and psychometric properties of the OSCE have been investigated and appear to be well established, particularly in general medical, surgery and internal medicine settings (Auewarkarul et al. 2005). In other words, raters can agree on what the test is measuring and can rate a candidate's performance consistently. While OSCEs are widely used in many disciplines, some areas, such as psychiatry, have not adopted them to anything like the same extent, and they have only recently been more widely introduced in undergraduate and postgraduate assessments worldwide (Auewarakul et al. 2005).

The development of OSCE examinations has been rapid over the last 30 years, often based upon roles played out by students with standard patients, real patients, actors, colleagues or even, as witnessed by one of us, a frantic hunt through the medical school for people who were in their offices, and 'free for a few minutes', who could play the part of a patient.

This kind of role-playing became such a dominant teaching device in clinical education as a result of conceptual and practical shifts in the training of counsellors and psychotherapists. It was reinforced by the advances in training brought about by audio and later video recording. Thus, this kind of training has come to have a well-established and respected place in the education of health professionals. While the origins of this approach can be most clearly seen in counselling and psychotherapy, in their present form role-playing exercises between students – or sometimes involving actors, stooges or real patients – have become a staple of education and assessment.

Trainees' OSCE performance may be used in a variety of ways to aid the pedagogic process. For example, formative feedback may be provided to examinees, perhaps as part of preparation for a further examination that counts towards their marks for the course. Additional purposes for OSCE assessments have included the evaluation of the effectiveness of curricular interventions, and to determine competency for obtaining qualifications or registration to practice. These exercises all assume that students who score higher on the OSCE checklist are better at communicating with patients (Mazor et al. 2005).

One variable that has been used widely as a measure of trainees' communication skills in such situations is the rating from the person playing the role of the patient. They may be asked about their level of satisfaction with the communication encounter, their level of ease with the student clinician, their sense that all the relevant aspects of their condition have been covered and so on. As Mazor et al. (2005) caution, however, the ratings from these standardized patients do not necessarily correspond to the ratings given by the examiners.

As well as these questions about the empirical consistency of the different kinds of ratings given in OSCE examinations there are a number of other issues that should be considered when exploring the suitability of role-playing. It is easy to be persuaded by the argument that practising skills, receiving feedback and evaluating students on their abilities in this respect is desirable. It is difficult to imagine wanting to be treated by a health professional who has not had sufficient practice at this kind of thing. However, we must be aware of what is lacking in such exercises.

OSCEs, and the kind of education for health care professionals in which they are used, often have a distinctively individual focus. They are often about undertaking the right communication behaviour. Examiners may assess the level of eye contact, the kinds of questions asked and yet this does not necessarily address the organizational factors which often constrain the real-life encounter. It is desirable to greet the client, introduce oneself and maintain culturally appropriate levels of eye contact (although given the variety of cultures this may be a virtually impossible repertoire to obtain). Yet once the training has been completed and the course passed, practitioners might find themselves working in an organization where the main priority is to process people as quickly as possible and the focus is on ensuring that electronic records or paper-based forms are completed properly. The complaint from patients that their doctor spends more time looking at the computer than he or she does looking at them was brought home to one of us (BB) recently upon hearing from a clinical colleague who had been to a seminar about record keeping where staff had been told that failure to complete the electronic patient record correctly was a dismissable offence! Assiduous attention to one's computer screen can perhaps be a valuable survival mechanism, but probably does not help one's diligently learned communication skills.

Education based on these kinds of role-plays and assessments does not generally have the ability to assess or encourage health care professionals in broader social interventions. We might for example assess a person's state of depression, yet initiating effective change in their social circumstances to alleviate their symptoms is beyond the scope of most OSCEs and indeed many health professionals. Looking at the picture of public health, skills and interventions that might be desirable at a family, community or societal level is much less easily assessed in these terms, and the focus of such education is not easily brought to bear on them.

The content of OSCEs, like that of much education for health care professionals tends to reinforce the received wisdom of what health care professionals should be doing. Determining their contents and the problems to be represented at an OSCE 'station' may represent educators' best guesses at the kinds of problems that students will later encounter in professional practice. Yet nevertheless they are contrived. Those in the role of patients are often carefully selected and trained so that a particular set of symptoms will be displayed. The extent to which they represent the often much more ambiguous problems in everyday life is often rather less carefully explored. They are thus vulnerable to the criticism that they are artificial.

The literature on exercises like these for clinicians in training and those in practice is generally positive about the effects. However, some cautionary notes must be sounded. Whereas outcomes are generally positive where they have been evaluated, and positive training effects yielded (Hulsman et al. 1999; Chan et al. 2003), positive effects of training were not noted in all the measures. Affective and interpersonal behaviour was noted to improve, but participants did not necessarily become more receptive or informative to patients. The better designed studies reported the fewest positive training effects (Hulsman et al. 1999; Chan et al. 2003).

Thus, despite the success of role-play-based education, and the frequently used OSCE style examination to assess trainee clinicians, there are key areas of health care activity that are generally left out of such activities, especially action at epidemiological, social or familial levels. The transferability of such training to practice may be offset by organizational constraints, and the more closely we examine its effects the less robust they might seem. Later in this volume we will explore some novel techniques based on other kinds of pedagogy which have some potential to address these other aspects of the communication learning process.

Models of the communication process in education for health care professionals

In terms of integrating communication into the curriculum for health care professionals, there have been a number of initiatives which have tried to achieve this. One of the better known is the Calgary-Cambridge framework for communication skills teaching (Kurtz et al. 1998; Silverman et al. 1998), which has been adopted by many UK medical schools (Spencer 2001). This is a structured approach to teaching communication in consultation settings which emphasizes the importance of integrating communication skills into the whole of the trainee practitioners' curriculum. If it is ghettoized into a module on communication skills, the fear is that the students will merely learn it for the course and not apply it elsewhere. Moreover, Kurtz et al. (2003) advocate that an approach that emphasizes communication skills is pursued through into work experience and employment, to ensure that the development of these skills is supported and consolidated, though as we have seen, sometimes in the workplace other considerations supervene and communication skills sometimes have to take second place to other more pressing matters like filling in record sheets.

In this section we will describe and offer some commentary on a number of different models of the communication process in health care. Many different models for training in consultation skills have been described (e.g. Pendleton et al. 1984; Gask et al. 1991) and some trainers and students will find themselves exposed to a number of different approaches. Our selection here does not seek to single out the examples used for criticism, nor to suggest they are better or more comprehensive than any others.

Heron's (1975) six-category intervention analysis

In the mid-1970s the humanistic psychologist, John Heron, developed a model of the array of interventions a doctor, counsellor or other therapist could use with the patient or client, which was intended to be both simple and comprehensive. Within an overall assumption that the professional is concerned for the patient's best interest the practitioner's interventions may fall into one or more of six categories:

1. *Prescriptive* – this involves giving advice or instructions, being critical or directive.
2. *Informative* – which might involve imparting new knowledge, instructing or interpreting.
3. *Confrontational* – which could involve challenging a restrictive attitude or behaviour, or giving direct feedback within a caring context.
4. *Cathartic* – that is, directed towards eliciting the release of emotion in the form of weeping, laughter, trembling or anger.
5. *Catalytic* – which includes encouraging the patient to discover and explore his or her own latent thoughts and feelings.
6. *Supportive* – as the name suggests, this intervention offers comfort and approval, and affirms the patient's intrinsic value.

Note that this is a functional model, inasmuch as the categories are all defined in terms of what they do or the effect they have. Each category is therefore intended to have a clear function within the total consultation. Interventions which might be intended as supportive might tend to come over as crass, patronizing or frankly sexist. A friend reported being told by a consultant psychiatrist, 'Aren't you pretty?' and on a subsequent appointment with the same man, accompanied by her mother was told, 'Don't you make a lovely family?' In the context of her quest to find a solution to some troubling neuropsychiatric symptoms she found these encounters offensive. Things, as the proverb has it, do not always turn out as planned, especially when values and ideas concerning gender roles have changed in the space of a generation.

Helman's (1981, 2001) folk model of illness

Cecil Helman, a medical anthropologist, with an interest in cultural factors in health and illness devised the following scheme based on his desire to understand why it was that people came to see health professionals. He proposed that a patient with a problem sees a doctor for answers to six questions:

1. What has happened?
2. Why has it happened?
3. Why to me?
4. Why now?
5. What would happen if nothing were done about it?
6. What should I do about it?

Again, as we can see, this is a model which emphasizes functions of the health care encounter and invites us to see the event from the point of view of the patient seeking answers to questions raised by pains, intimations of illness or a failure of his or her ability to 'cope'. The emphasis then is on what the client or patient is seeking to gain.

Seven activities: Pendleton et al. (1984)

A somewhat different approach was taken by Pendleton and colleagues who described seven activities which together make up a set of aims that may be pursued in a clinical consultation. As a result of their observations, Pendleton and co-workers identified the tasks as:

1. To define the reason for the patient's attendance, including
    (a) the nature and history of the problems
    (b) their aetiology
    (c) the patient's ideas, concerns and expectations
    (d) the effects of the problems.

2. To consider other problems:
    (a) continuing problems
    (b) at-risk factors.

3. With the patient, to choose an appropriate action for each problem.

4. To achieve a shared understanding of the problems with the patient.

5. To involve the patient in the management and encourage him/her to accept appropriate responsibility.

6. To use time and resources appropriately
    (a) in the consultation
    (b) in the long term.

7. To establish and maintain a relationship with the patient which helps to achieve the other tasks.

These have been widely used and taught as appropriate aims for the consultation. Looking at them, one can readily see that they are of a rather different order than the previous two approaches. There is a somewhat different emphasis in that the first item is actively heuristic; it involves treating the patient and the problem as if they were unknown territories to be discovered. There are management and resource considerations built in too, inasmuch as there are exhortations to use time and resources appropriately. These items in Pendleton and colleagues's scheme have been used extensively as a means of assessing trainee practitioners' performance. They may yield an improved experience for the patient, but they also embody issues that, for example, a doctor may need to know to manage his or her practice effectively.

The triaxial model (Working Party of the Royal College of General Practitioners 1972)

In the early 1970s the Royal College of General Practitioners highlighted the need for doctors to address patient problems in terms of the three 'axes' of physical, psychological and social issues. This was intended to reflect contemporary thinking about the consultation – and health care more generally – that it should ideally reflect the interaction of these three issues. This was also reflected in the 'biopsychosocial model' popularized by Engel (1977). The motivating idea was to discourage doctors from thinking purely in organic terms and consider the patient's emotional, family, social and environmental circumstances, all of which were increasingly suspected to have a profound effect on health.

Calgary-Cambridge approach to communication skills teaching (Kurtz and Silverman 1996)

In the 1990s as concerns about communication skills – or the lack of them – in health professionals reached fever pitch, Suzanne Kurtz and Jonathan Silverman developed a model of the consultation, encapsulated within a practical teaching tool called the Calgary-Cambridge Observation Guides. These Guides define the content of a communication skills curriculum by delineating and structuring the skills that have been shown by research and theory to aid doctor–patient communication. The guides also intended to provide a concise and accessible summary for facilitators and learners alike which can also be used as an *aide memoire* during teaching sessions. The structure of the consultation proposed by these guides is as follows:

1. Initiating the session which can involve
    (a) establishing initial rapport
    (b) identifying the reason(s) for the consultation.

2. Gathering information which comprises
    (a) exploration of problems
    (b) understanding the patient's perspective
    (c) providing structure to the consultation.

3. Building the relationship:
    (a) developing rapport
    (b) involving the patient.

4. Explanation and planning:
    (a) providing the correct amount and type of information

(b) aiding accurate recall and understanding
(c) achieving a shared understanding: incorporating the patient's perspective
(d) planning: shared decision making.

5. Closing the session.

As we can see, this summary of the scheme by Kurtz and Silverman proceeds sequentially. Rather like the consultation itself, one can almost see it on an evaluation sheet with tick boxes for the examiner to identify whether each stage has been passed through satisfactorily.

Many of these schemes have been built on the assumption that what we are trying to do with the encounter is identify the nature and causes of the problem, with a view to going on to agree an intervention or treatment. Of course, this isn't always what happens. Many health care encounters, especially those undertaken by people other than primary care physicians, may be more geared to monitoring the progress of an already known condition, or be concerned with undertaking part of a prolonged series of interventions. There is a distinct sense that, with many of these schemes, they are designed to facilitate an efficient and impeccably polite screening of the clients so that the cause of the problem can be identified and addressed by whatever means are available. What are far less evident in the literature are models of how students can be taught to care for people who have chronic conditions requiring multiple consultations.

The communication skills that are considered desirable in trainee practitioners have been further itemized and assessed in a scheme devised by Walters et al. (2005: 294) who described the following series of assessment tasks they devised for their students. This is designed for students being trained in mental health, but we can see that a number of aspects of this series can be found in many other branches of health care:

1. *History-taking 'interactive' stations* Here the student is asked to take a focused psychiatric history on a mental health topic. For example, they may be asked to take a brief history and make an assessment of suicidal risk in a person who has deliberately self-harmed, take an alcohol history or take a history from a person presenting with panic attacks.

2. *Communication skills 'interactive' stations* These had two forms: talking to a relative about a diagnosis and explaining a treatment option to a patient. In the first type the student had to respond to the concerns or questions posed by a relative of someone recently diagnosed with a mental health disorder, such as schizophrenia or Alzheimer's disease. In the second the student was asked to counsel a patient about a treatment option, for example different 'talking therapies' for depression or starting a new psychiatric drug therapy.

3. *Telephone communication with colleague* Students were asked to role-play the duty psychiatrist on call, giving telephone advice to another health professional (played by the examiner). Typical scenarios included a GP ringing about a potentially at-risk patient with psychosis or a charge nurse from a

general medical ward asking for advice on management of an elderly patient with acute confusion.

4. *Video mental state examination* Two video stations were included in each OSCE. Students watch a 4-minute video clip of a real or simulated patient and are asked to record a written mental state examination. The video recordings were made with consent specifically for use in teaching and the OSCE, mainly with in-patients on the wards over the preceding year being interviewed by psychiatric specialist training registrars. The clinical problems were mainly psychosis, but also included severe depression and cognitive impairment.

5. *Written case vignette* Students were asked to answer problem-orientated questions based on an evolving case scenario in a short answer format. A wide range of clinical problems and patients were included in this format.

6. *Written problem-orientated vignette with visual prompt* Similar to the standard written case vignette, these stations used visual prompts as well as case scenarios to stimulate the students. Examples of prompts used include a brief video clip of someone with Parkinsonism from his anti-psychotic treatment, a blood result showing toxic lithium levels or a weight chart for someone with an eating disorder.

What is interesting here is that the set of skills identified as important has been extended to include considerably more than an initial consultation. It addresses concerns that health professionals do not communicate well with relatives by explicitly including this. It also assesses clear and effective communication with colleagues, addressing anecdotal concerns expressed to one of us by a clinical colleague who said that when he spoke to personnel on 'his ward' of mental health patients by phone, he sometimes couldn't tell whether he was talking to a colleague or a patient, such was the mumbling and confusion on the part of junior doctors. Nurses, he opined were 'a bit more brisk'.

Having trained the students according to the schemes above and assessed them on their OSCEs, Wilkinson and Fontaine (2002) raise the issue of how we should assess them. In developing marking schedules a number of factors can be taken into account. There is some debate as to how useful it is to include ratings from the patients. Wilkinson and Fontaine's standard patients told the authors they liked to be consulted. However, these patients are not experienced in student assessment and their training is more concerned with how they present their symptoms and is geared to ensuring that all the students get a similar presentation. This leads to a dilemma. On the one hand their opinions might be considered 'too subjective' and 'unreliable' or, in contrast, their very naïveté might give them a certain value as being rather like the lay-people who will be the ultimate recipients of the students' skills. Many educators and researchers have used standardized patients in assessing clinical skills. In rating the performance of the student, the standardized patient is often asked, for example, whether a preagreed list of topics has been covered. In some cases then, if the patient does the assessment, an examiner may not need to be present and this may help eliminate some of the variability in patient behaviour, thus giving the students a more standardized case to evaluate (Tamblyn et al. 1991). A good deal of the training such patients receive is geared to the reduction of this variability. In this way the correlation between patients' ratings of students' performance and ratings by other examiners can be increased. This convergence can be increased further by the use of checklists of the same attributes to be completed by patients and examiners (MacRae et al. 1995). Thus, the technical dilemmas of assessment can be reduced. Even if it is a little contrived, the application of a progressive approach to standardization can resolve what might otherwise be a divergence in ratings and an internally consistent system of marking can be achieved.

Despite the achievement of consistency, there may be more issues to unpack in this increasingly protocol-driven approach to education for clinicians. Robinson et al. (2003) remind us that learning is about considerably more than the mechanical practising of 'skills'; activity and reflection are further integral parts of the learning process (Kolb 1984). In the sense meant by Robinson et al. (2003), 'activity' is connected with the awareness of experience. The processes of reflection and awareness are not generally foregrounded in schemes of skills or typologies of the clinical encounter used in training, but to many theorists of education they are vital. For example, Schön (1983) argues that expert practitioners are able to 'reflect in action'. In other words they do so 'on the fly' as they exercise their expertise, so that their performance may be geared to the circumstances. This process is often subliminal and may appear to work on automatic pilot. Some clinical practitioners sometimes speak of 'brain stem memory' for a skill that is very well learned and automated.

At higher levels of challenge the practitioner may need to pause and think, perhaps deferring a decision until a course of action has been consciously thought through. From observation of expert performance, Schön (1983) also relates how an intuition that 'something does not fit' does not necessarily interrupt the practitioner's flow, but may be resolved on later reflection. These kinds of conception of the practice of skill do not lend themselves so well to a neat typology and a list of items that examiners, standardized patients and students can check off on a worksheet. Related to this is the insistence some theorists of the health care process have on the importance of 'lived experience', supporting the development of a patient- orientated disposition. Duncan et al. (2003) argue that such a focus is crucial to all involved in the practice of health care and is intimately connected with the idea of the 'good health care practitioner'.

Looking at the larger picture: liberatory education for professionals in training

In trying to contextualize the learning process, the principles of Paulo Freire, a Brazilian educator, are perhaps relevant. The ethics of everyday communicative interventions and the interest in lived experience have some resonance with his work. Freire's (1990) method was intended to help participants in an educational intervention discover the truth of their own experience, how they got where they are, and how they can act in the world to facilitate change. Freire's methods were considered innovative and sought to use the knowledge and experience of the participants and learner rather than assuming that the participant is an empty vessel to be filled with the knowledge of the 'expert' teacher. Now in the circumstances we are talking about, where novice, inexperienced students are trying to learn consultation skills, using role-played or standardized patients and under the tutelage of staff in medical or nursing schools who probably know more than they do, this process might seem a little far fetched. After all, the experienced clinicians and tutors know more than the students? Researchers have diligently examined different techniques so that we are now confident of what students can do to maximize the disclosure of diagnostically relevant information and yield higher patient satisfaction ratings. If only they would learn how to do it!

However, issues relating to virtues, ethics and radical pedagogies are relevant here. After all, students arrive in these training programmes already knowing about how to have conversations with people. Yet in all too many cases their pre-existing fluency becomes, with the benefit of training, awkward, stilted and self-conscious so that in some cases it is almost painful to watch. This prompts the question as to what has happened to the knowledge and humane ambitions they had prior to training, about wanting to help people and do something that makes a difference.

It is through watching this spectacle that Freire's approach, which focuses on the liberation and empowerment of participants (Hope et al. 1992), has suggested itself to us. Freire (1990) envisioned the education process as one in which learners act not as recipients, but as knowing subjects achieving a deepening awareness both of the sociocultural reality that shapes their lives and of their capacity to transform that reality. Thus we are mindful in our own work of what we can do that adds to the knowledge and power of students rather than detracts from it. The question is one of how to increase awareness and the ability, as the cliché has it, to tap one's power. This may include overcoming a sense of inadequacies, recognizing the changes one is able to effect, and understanding one's position in a social context (Werner and Bower 1982). When we have asked students in seminar groups about the process of communicating with clients and how to deal with the need to elicit diagnostically relevant information and make the client feel good about the consultation, even relatively naïve students have come up with pretty much the same solutions as the experts after years of research. Even the most hesitant student knows a good deal about what to do. The problem, which we have yet to entirely resolve, is how to build on that knowledge.

If students are able to use the knowledge they bring to the encounter as well as the guidelines the have learned about 'good communication' we can sometimes see a 'step change' in their ability to identify the problems. Such an example comes from Duncan et al. (2003: 188):

> I was with the student and he was taking a history of this guy who'd presented with headaches, basically. He was asking lots of questions about, 'What exactly are the symptoms? Are you getting dizzy?', whatever. And he was getting nowhere, and then suddenly he started off on a whole different line of questioning. About what was going on at home. Was the guy working?, etc. And it basically turned out that this guy was suffering from stress. And after, when I was going through it with the student and asking him why he'd

changed his questions, he said that he'd suddenly noticed that the bloke's eyes were red. That he looked exhausted, and that somehow this was more to do with what was going on in the rest of his life and not just to do with the headaches. [Philip, GP tutor]

The proliferation of guidelines and protocols for clinical effectiveness may also seriously inhibit professionals from fully realizing such an imaginative way of working (Hart et al. 2003: 488). The challenge for educators and practitioners themselves is to find a means of addressing their own education and clients' problems, which allows us to build on the strengths and knowledge they bring to the educational setting. These are often many and various, including strengths at communicating, passing on information and offering comfort outside the clinical setting which often seem to be lost when they cross the threshold into the consulting room. In the next chapter therefore we will be dealing with some of the ways in which this ability can be enhanced rather than eroded, and make some novel suggestions concerning the education of the future health care workforce.

References

Auewarkarul, C., Downing, S.M., Praditsuwan, R. and Jaturatamrong, U. (2005) Item analysis to improve reliability for an internal medicine undergraduate OSCE, *Advances in Health Sciences Education*, 10: 105–13.

Bloor, M. and McIntosh, J. (1990) Surveillance and concealment: a comparison of techniques of client resistance in therapeutic communities and health visiting, in S. Cunningham-Burley and N. McKeganey (eds) *Readings in Medical Sociology*. London: Routledge.

Booth K., Maguire P. and Hillier V.F. (1999) Measurement of communication skills in cancer care: myth or reality? *Journal of Advanced Nursing*, 30: 1073–9.

Bowles, N., Macintosh, C. and Torn, A. (2001) Nurses' communication skills: an evaluation of the impact of solution-focused communication training, *Journal of Advanced Nursing*, 36(3): 347–54.

Butterwick, S. and Benjamin, A. (2006) The road to employability through personal development: a critical analysis of the silences and ambiguities of the British Columbia (Canada) Life Skills Curriculum, *International Journal of Lifelong Education*, 25(1): 75–86.

Chan, C.S.Y., Wun, Y.T., Cheung, A. et al. (2003) Communication skill of general practitioners: Any room for improvement? How much can it be improved? *Medical Education*, 37: 514–26.

Contu, A., Grey, C. and Ortenblad, A. (2003) Against learning, *Human Relations*, 56(8): 931–52.

Crute, V.C., Hargie, O.D.W. and Ellis, R.A.F. (1989) An evaluation of a communication skills course for health visitor students, *Journal of Advanced Nursing*, 14: 546–52.

Dearing, R. (1997) *Higher Education in the Learning Society*. London: Stationery Office.

Duncan, P., Cribb, A. and Stephenson, A. (2003) Developing 'the good health care practitioner': clues from a study in medical education, *Learning in Health and Social Care*, 2(4): 181–90.

Eastwood, J.B., Conroy, R.E., Naicker, S., West, P., Tutt, R.C. and Plange-Rhule, J. (2005) Loss of health professionals from sub-Saharan Africa: the pivotal role of the UK, *Lancet*, 365: 1893–900.

Edwards, J. and Popay, J. (1994) Contradictions of support and self help: views from providers of community health and social services to families with young children, *Health and Social Care in the Community*, 2: 31–40.

Engel, G.L. (1977) The need for a new medical model: the challenge for biomedicine, *Science*, 196: 129–36.

Fairclough, N. (1989) *Language and Power.* London: Longman.

Fairclough, N. (2003) *Analyzing Discourse and Text: Textual Analysis for Social Research.* London: Routledge.

Fielding, R.G. and Llewelyn, S.P. (1979) Communication training in nursing may damage your health and your enthusiasm: some warnings, *Journal of Advanced Nursing*, 12: 281–90.

Fraser, N. (1997) *Justice Interruptus: Critical Reflections on the 'Postsocialist' Condition.* London: Routledge.

Freire, P. (1990) *Pedagogy of the Oppressed.* New York: Continuum.

Furedi, F. (2004) *Therapy Culture: Cultivating Vulnerability in an Uncertain Age.* London: Routledge.

Gask, L., Boardman, A.P. and Standart, S. (1991) Teaching communication skills: a problem-based approach, *Postgraduate Education in General Practice*, 2: 7–15.

Gorovitz, S. (1994) Is caring a viable component of health care? *Health Care Analysis*, 2: 129–33.

Harden, R., Stevenson, M., Downie, W. and Wilson, G. (1975). Assessment of clinical competence using objective structured examinations, *British Medical Journal*, 1: 447–51.

Hart, A., Lockey, R., Henwood, F., Pankhurst, F., Hall, V. and Sommerville, F. (2001) *Addressing Inequalities in Health: New Directions in Midwifery Education and Practice.* London: English National Board for Nursing, Midwifery and Health Visiting.

Hart, A., Hall, V. and Henwood, F. (2003) Helping health and social care professionals to develop an 'inequalities imagination': a model for use in education and practice, *Journal of Advanced Nursing*, 41(5): 480–9.

Helman, C.G. (1981) Disease versus illness in general practice, *Journal of the Royal College of General Practitioners*, 31: 548–62.

Helman, C.G. (2001) *Culture, Health and Illness*, 4th edn. London: Arnold.

Heron, J. (1975) *A Six Category Intervention Analysis: Human Potential Research Project.* Brighton: University of Surrey.

Hope, A., Timmel, S. and Hodzi, C. (1992) *Training for Transformation* (Books 1–3). Gweru, Zimbabwe: Mambo Press.

Hulsman, R.L., Ros, W.J.G., Winnubst, J.A.M. and Bensing, J.M. (1999) Teaching clinically experienced physicians communication skills. A review of evaluation studies, *Medical Education*, 33: 655–68.

Kolb, D. (1984) *Experiential Learning.* Englewood Cliffs, NJ: Prentice Hall.

Kurtz, S. and Silverman, J. (1996) The Calgary-Cambridge Observation Guides: an aid to defining the curriculum and organizing the teaching in communication training programmes, *Medical Education*, 30: 83–9.

Kurtz, S., Silverman, J. and Draper, J. (1998) *Teaching and Learning Communication Skills in Medicine.* Oxford: Radcliffe Medical Press.

Kurtz, S., Silverman, J., Benson, J. and Draper, J. (2003) Marrying content and process in clinical method teaching: enhancing the Calgary-Cambridge Guides, *Academic Medicine*, 78(8): 802–9.

McCue, J.D. (1982) The effects of stress on physicians and their medical practice, *New England Journal of Medicine*, 306: 458–63.

MacLean, I. (1994) Doctor Rabelais's 500 year old prescription, *British Medical Journal*, 308: 803–4.

MacRae, H.M., Vu, N.V., Graham, B., Word-Sims, M., Colliver, J.A. and Robbs, R.S. (1995) Comparing checklists and databases with physicians' ratings as measures of students' history and physical examination skills, *Academic Medicine*, 70: 313–17.

Mazor, K.M., Ockene, J.K., Rogers, H.J., Carlin, M.M. and Quirk, M.E. (2005) The relationship between checklist scores on a communication OSCE and analogue patients' perceptions of communication, *Advances in Health Sciences Education*, 10: 37–51.

Nagano, H. (2001) Empathic understanding: constructing an evaluation scale from the micro-counseling approach, *Nursing and Health Sciences*, 2: 17–27.

Nelson-Jones, R. (2002) Are there universal human being skills? *Counselling Psychology Quarterly*, 15(2): 115–19.

Newton, T., Handy, J. and Fineman, S. (1996) *Managing Stress: Emotion and Power at Work*. London: Sage.

The Observer (2006) Let's decide what we really want from universities (leader), 19 February.

Opengart, R. and Short, D.C. (2002) Free agent learners: the new career model and its impact on human resource development, *International Journal of Lifelong Education*, 21(3): 220–33.

Pendleton, D., Schofield, T., Tate, P. and Havelock, P. (1984) *The Consultation: An Approach to Learning and Teaching*. Oxford: Oxford University Press.

Peplau, H.E. (1952) *Interpersonal Relations in Nursing*. New York: G.P. Putnam's Sons.

Robinson, P., Purves, I. and Wilson, R. (2003) Learning support for the consultation: information support and decision support should be placed in an educational framework, *Medical Education*, 37: 429–33.

Schön, D. (1983) *The Reflective Practitioner: How Professionals Think in Action*. London: Maurice Temple Smith.

Silverman, J.D., Kurtz, S.M. and Draper, J. (1998) *Skills for Communicating with Patients*. Oxford: Radcliffe Medical Press.

Spencer, J. (2001) Education for communication: much already known, so much more to understand, *Medical Education*, 35: 188–90.

Stewart, M., Brown, J.B., Donner, A., McWhinney, I.R., Oates, J. and Weston, W.W. (2000) The impact of patient-centered care on outcomes, *Journal of Family Practice*, 49: 796–804.

Suikkala, A. and Leino-Kilpi, H. (2001) Nursing student–patient relationships: a review of the literature from 1984 to 1998, *Journal of Advanced Nursing*, 33: 42–50.

Tamblyn, R.M., Klass, D.J., Schnabl, G.K. and Kopelow, M.L. (1991) Sources of unreliability and bias in standardized patient rating, *Teaching and Learning in Medicine*, 3: 74–85.

Walters, K., Osborn, P. and Raven, P. (2005) The development, validity and reliability of a multimodality objective structured clinical examination in psychiatry, *Medical Education*, 39: 292–8.

Weatherall, D.J. (1994) The inhumanity of medicine, *British Medical Journal*, 309: 527.

Weinberg, A. and Creed, F. (2000) Stress and psychiatric disorder in health care professionals and hospital staff, *Lancet*, 355: 533–7.

Werner, D. and Bower, B. (1982) *Helping Health Workers Learn*. Palo Alto, CA: Hesperian Foundation.

Wilkinson S., Bailey K., Aldridge J. and Roberts A. (1999) A longitudinal evaluation of a communication skills programme, *Palliative Medicine*, 13: 341–8.

Wilkinson, T.J. and Fontaine, S. (2002) Patients' global ratings of student competence. Unreliable contamination or gold standard? *Medical Education*, 36: 1117–21.

Working Party of the Royal College of General Practitioners (1972) *The Triaxial Model of the Consultation*. London: Royal College of General Practitioners.

Young, M. (1970) A general practitioner considers nursing education, in M. Innnis (ed.) *Nursing Education in a Changing Society*. Toronto: University of Toronto Press.

7 New approaches to the teaching of communication: data-driven learning and experiential education

Education for the future

In this chapter we will consider some of the possibilities for teaching students and professionals about health care communication that might be explored more fully in the future and which, we believe, will lead to a more fully evidence-based educational experience for practitioners. A closer integration of teaching, learning and research will equip practitioners more appropriately, so they can see their work as a continuous process of enquiry rather than something that you learn about in college or on days of training offered as part of continuing professional development programmes.

So far in our exploration of teaching and learning in health care communication we have been proceeding as if this were a relatively easy process to conceptualize. Much of the material we have reviewed so far is predicated on the assumption that the trainee health care professional's communication will be improved as they learn skills that enable them to interact more effectively with clients. In this chapter we will try something different: presenting some of the newer and alternative approaches that have been attempted to facilitate learning the languages and skills of communication in health care contexts. In order to do this we must necessarily reflect a little more on what it is that learning and teaching are trying to achieve and how they might best be understood. This kind of reflection is perhaps appropriate given that the central focus of so much of the literature on health care communication has been upon getting students to communicate with patients so as to elicit the right diagnostic information. This has allowed a number of key assumptions of the teaching and learning process to remain under-explored.

Despite the enthusiasm with which educators and professional bodies governing health care seized on the idea of training in communication, critical or questioning voices have frequently been raised. From the inception of the present-day concern with health care communication about a decade or so ago, a number of concerns were mooted. For example, the use of role-play was not thought be appropriate for all cultural and ethnic groups, and the styles of communicative practice preferred in most western approaches to interpersonal encounters in medicine were noted not to be equally appropriate in other parts of the world (Curr 1994).

Let us begin this chapter therefore by trying to unpack the meaning of teaching and learning, and having done that, we can move on to try to understand it differently and explore the other kinds of transformations which students, teachers and patients are supposed to undergo during the communicative process.

The nature of learning and teaching in health care communication

To begin with, we can readily identify some straightforward and uncontentious attempts to understand what learning is. In many accounts, a student-centred approach is signalled towards the teaching and learning process. For example it is sometimes said that the central purpose of teaching is to help someone learn (Pratt 1998; D'Eon 2004); learning is the goal and the reason for our instructional efforts (D'Eon 2004: 604). The American Psychological Association defines learning as a relatively durable change in an individual. In this formulation, to learn means to change, to be able to do or think or feel something new and different to some useful purpose.

The learning process was further subdivided into a classic typology by Bloom (1956) which yielded three generally accepted broad areas or domains of human behaviour in which learning was believed to take place: *thinking* (cognitive domain), *doing* (psychomotor) and *feeling* (affective). Added to this list, especially relevant to learning communication practices in health care settings is a fourth domain that encompasses relating in groups (social/relational) (Mackway-Jones and Walker 1999). As D'Eon (2004: 604) puts it, what we are aiming for in education for health care professionals in interdisciplinary settings is for 'learners to adopt effective and successful strategies and where applicable shed and/or modify less effective ones in all domains of learning'. In addition, the process of learning is frequently conceived of as being related to connections made by the learner between different areas and issues of importance to him or her: 'Sound knowledge is based on interconnections ... Understanding is itself the realization that what is separate in ignorance is connected in knowing' (Biggs 1999: 73). This interconnectedness is developed by building on what is already known. In educational settings this can be enhanced by making the training task similar to the target transfer task (Biggs 1999; Custers and Boshuizen 2002).

In connection with students' development in the health care professions, the tradition of experiential learning has a long history in health care as doctors and nurses traditionally learned their craft practically on the job. It is comparatively recently in historical terms that the training in these disciplines has become a largely academic matter, based in universities. Indeed, it has been suggested that this has allowed universities rather than the professions themselves to seize control of training.

From the point of view of seeking to understand what goes on in teaching and learning, the experiential on-the-job learning in health care involves some distinctive assumptions about the role of the learner and teacher. Often, the philosophies of experiential and practice-based learning assume that students should have 'ownership over their own learning process and their right to make decisions about the direction it takes' (Dewar and Walker 1999: 1462). In this way, they are assumed to be able to be self-directing and more autonomous learners.

In the literature on training, learning and instructional practice, many accounts of the processes concerned derive from work in military or industrial contexts. We might learn how novices master the art of operating machinery, or how air traffic controllers monitor many different ongoing tasks using the assistive technologies of the control tower. These accounts then come from the occupations and industries where the processes are relatively easy to observe by the informed inquirer, and originate in contexts where safety is critical and investment in training analysis has been high, leaving researchers and educators with the leisure to write up their findings in the technical literature. Some education in health care has yielded a similar literature, especially marked by the investment in training for medical doctors. However, there are many ways in which the kinds of training in health care and its overall objectives are different from the often highly specific goals in business or military contexts. Health care education goals are diverse and rarely defined concretely (Shipengrover and James 1999).

Integrating experience and learning theory

As we have noted training often aims to make students technically proficient and enable them to master the mechanisms of disease. Yet they are also increasingly expected to be skilled, compassionate communicators with patients and their families, to keep themselves abreast of new research for evidence-based practice, and to investigate themselves where puzzling questions in health care emerge. This vision is filled with contradictory values. Furthermore, it may take some time to pass before educational goals are actualized in student behaviour, with changes sometimes taking a generation or more to flush through the system. Health care education is a long-term investment with multiple beneficiaries who are not always identified as stakeholders at the outset. As Shipengrover and James (1999) note, these vague and contradictory visions can lead to difficulty in characterizing and measuring the outcomes of education in health care.

There have been a number of contemporary initiatives where training and education have involved students in being encouraged to take on a small caseload of clients whom they can get to know and help through episodes of illness (O'Keeffe et al. 2001; Wilkinson et al. 2002). This experiential education builds on some of the principles of Paulo Freire which we saw in the previous chapter. In addition to this, there are initiatives to extend the process of communication into new areas of the health care process. Lindwall et al. (2003) describe the use of communication innovations such as attempts to engage with the patient's feelings and thoughts at the time they are scheduled for operations, and conclude that 'perioperative conversations' between clients and nurses have beneficial outcomes for clients. These kinds of innovations mean that the process of education has to be re-thought and re-evaluated.

Following the generative work of Drefyus and Dreyfus in trying to characterize expertise, a number of authors have attempted to distinguish the nature of expertise as applied to health care practice. According to authors such as Bransford et al. (1999) or Dunphy and Williamson (2004) expertise in practical health care contexts has six important characteristics.

First, experts can recognize features and meaningful patterns of information that are not noticed by novices. Expert clinicians may be able to use their communication skills to elicit key pieces of information from a patient's description which enable them to recognize regularities that can be combined to yield diagnoses that would not be identified immediately by a novice clinician.

Second, experts have usually acquired a great deal of 'content knowledge', about the field in which they practice which is organized so as to reflect a structured thematic understanding of their subject matter.

Third, expert knowledge is not simply a list of isolated facts or propositions but instead, knowledge is 'conditionalized' so as to reflect contexts of applicability dependent on sets of circumstances.

Fourth, experts are able to fluently and flexibly retrieve important aspects of their knowledge with little attentional effort.

Fifth, although experts – including expert communicators – know their craft and their parent discipline thoroughly, this does not necessarily make them good teachers. This aspect may however be enhanced if the experts concurrently develop expertise in teaching or coaching.

Sixth, and finally, experts can strategically vary their level of flexibility in their approach to new situations.

Knowledge acquisition in a social context

Communicative action and communication learning always take place in some kind of social context. This context can be especially important if it facilitates or inhibits learning or if it presents problems which limit the scope and effectiveness of the communication which can take place. In this section therefore we will deal with some educational efforts to understand that context, both from the point of view of those learning and from the point of view of people whose opportunities to communicate are restricted by circumstances.

The social context of learning has been seen as important by many educators, and has also been seen as a resource that can facilitate the learning process. Being able to observe colleagues at work, and participate in the local work culture of practice and the learning communities of the workplace, enhance this process. Thus, advice to learn by watching more experienced colleagues (Patvardhan 2005), or the literature on the value of learning communities in workplaces (Eraut 1994) and the value attached to informal learning all address this issue. Communitarian, milieu-based learning is therefore important as well as anything that can be formally learned in the classroom.

This also ties in with the notion of situated learning (Lave and Wenger 1991) and distributed cognition (Salomon 1993). A good deal of the study of learning has proceeded as if it involved individual cognitive processes which were 'possessed and residing in the heads of individuals' (Salomon 1993: xii). By contrast the study of distributed cognition has looked to the tools and social relations 'outside' people's heads. They are not only 'sources of stimulation and guidance but are actually vehicles of thought ... It is not just the "person-solo" who learns, but the "person-plus", the whole system of interrelated factors' ((p. xiii). In other words, people think in and through relationships with others and use a variety of socially and culturally available tools. Different cognitions will emerge in different situations. In this respect the study of socialized cognition draws us back to Pierre Bourdieu's notions of habitus and doxa which we encountered in Chapter 1. Bourdieu (1984, 1986, 1991, 1998) delineated the processes by which individuals and groups use varying degrees of cultural knowledge symbolically as cultural capital for personal advantage in ways that stratify communities. Although not yet used extensively to study communication in health care as such, Bourdieu's perspective has much potential to aid understanding of the nature of organizational and cultural processes in health care in a new light.

A further aspect of the role of context in people's experiences of communication in health care situations is the involvement of power. Once we start thinking about context, it rapidly becomes apparent that it is not a level playing field. The contexts of learning and the contexts of practice are often not a 'level playing field'. Indeed, collaborative learning of the kind we mentioned earlier often seeks to resist cultural reproduction what Pierre Bourdieu (1986) identifies as the scarcely conscious transmission and adoption of arbitrary values, styles, tastes and discursive forms privileged by groups or classes in power.

In this context, a further effort to improve the education of health care professionals which has significant implications for communicative practice comes from educators who seek to develop in their students an awareness of the role of power and inequality in clients' lives. This is understood by many radical educators and practitioners to be important since the powerlessness associated with social inequality is a psychosocial risk factor for increased morbidity and mortality (Wallerstein 1992) such that people who do not have the means to access services and information are more likely to suffer illnesses and injury such as infectious diseases, injuries from violence, and chronic illness. Thus, a focus on inequality and empowerment to overcome this has appealed to theorists and educators in health education, medicine, nursing and especially social work as a strategy for enhancing the wellbeing of people whose health is affected by social conditions (Miller 1992; Connor et al. 1999). It offers the possibility of enabling people to alleviate some of the longer term problems affecting their health, rather than merely treating the symptoms when they become unbearable. In the UK, government policy seeking to reduce the number of children growing up in poverty, or seeking to combat 'social exclusion' is founded on similar premises. In assisting students to gain an awareness of these issues Hart et al. (2003) discuss trying to give students an 'inequalities imagination' which will allow practitioners to address clients' needs and effectively challenge structural inequalities in a flexible way. The inequalities, disadvantages and oppressions which limit clients' health are many and various and may even emanate from the health services themselves, so a flexible imaginative approach is foregrounded. To illustrate this, consider the following anecdote related by a colleague who worked as a mental health support worker:

> There was this one bloke I worked with and he'd been out of hospital for a few months, maybe six months at the most and the one thing I noticed one day was how thin his arms were and then it turned out he wasn't eating and I looked at him, he was soaked, I mean from the waist down, and he'd been lounging around on the sofa and not getting up to the toilet, it just was all

soaking through, so then he'd got bed sores, obviously, and like nappy rash but really deep. It wasn't his fault he was just so crippled by the drugs he was taking and he just couldn't feel it, but then he told me he wasn't going to the toilet because the voices he was hearing, well they were worse in the bathroom.

In this case, the difficulties experienced by the client originated from a variety of problems, some of which perhaps might be iatrogenic, as well as the problems resulting from his hearing voices which had prompted his initial contact with health professionals and his treatment with antipsychotic medication. In our colleague's opinion this has resulted in the lethargy responsible for his loss of continence, and incidentally for the cigarette burns which pock-marked his fingers. The surrounding squalour, including the dirty, threadbare carpets whose grime came perilously close to the sores on his feet, and the mould that was eating its way through the peeling wallpaper in his flat served only to compound the sense of desolation. The inequalities facing clients then are often multiple and intersecting, relating to arcane benefits systems, approaches to care which focus on symptoms rather than the person and their circumstances, overlain by the blight of poverty and 'disempowerment'. Whereas the problems described here are all too often difficult to disentangle, even for those knowledgeable and skilled in medicine, social care or the legal system, the 'inequalities imagination' provides a way of grasping the nature of the problems in the first place.

The ideas of powerlessness and its opposite, empowerment, have been topics of investigation since the 1950s in social science and political theory (Wallerstein 1992). This concern has informed thinkers in the health care disciplines too. For example Abbott et al. (1997: 270) say that:

> Most mental health professionals agree that individuals who are empowered, who believe that they can influence or change their lives, are much better adjusted and self-confident than those who see themselves as victims ... empowered individuals are generally satisfied, motivated, and independent. According to Bate, 'empowerment means becoming powerful enough to accomplish your own goals and spreading the power you possess so that other people become able to accomplish their goals as well.'

As Connor et al. (1999) argue, this 'spreading' power tends to move outward to affect others in the manner of ripples on a pond, rather than remaining as a power that dominates, or which resides in a dominant source. According to Arbetter (cited in Abbott et al. 1997), empowerment involves decreasing the feeling of helplessness and increasing in the belief that one has the ability to bring about change. Empowerment enhances 'cooperation, creativity, communication, motivation, and feelings of competency and success ... [which] may have far-reaching consequences' (p. 270).

In the past two decades, investigations of powerlessness (also referred to as alienation, victim-blaming and learned helplessness) in health education, nursing and other fields have developed a picture of the relationship between powerlessness and disease. When groups of people are alienated from the dominant culture of their society, the subjective and objective control they have over their lives is decreased and this appears to constitute a risk factor for a variety of health problems (Wallerstein 1992). Conversely, many theorists and researchers see empowerment as being a key factor in the enhancement of wellbeing and of effective communication between clients, practitioners and policymakers, and advocate the realignment of health and social care to reflect this. Prilleltensky (2005: 59) says: 'Reactive, individual, alienating, and deficit-based approaches that foster patienthood instead of health, citizenship, and democracy have dominated the field of health and human services for decades'.

These concerns, that health care actively contributes to the disadvantage of some already marginalized groups in society, have led to a number of initiatives designed to alleviate the problem. In the UK the government at the time of writing has invested in combating what it calls social exclusion. In education for health and social care professionals there have been many attempts to adjust training and models of practice so that they can become liberatory rather than oppressive. These attempts have included efforts to try to make practice 'anti-oppressive' or 'anti-discriminatory' and have often tried to initiate some affective change on the part of the students so as to make them more willing to challenge the inequalities and exclusions that lead to their clients being in a dire situation.

Anti-discriminatory and anti-oppressive models of practice are often defined in very similar ways and neither is without critics. The precise relevance and practicality of these issues in training and education for human services professionals has been hotly debated for over a decade. Preston-Shoot (1995), in particular, maintains that anti-oppressive practice is more radical than anti-discriminatory practice in that it tries to challenge both structural and individual aspects of inequality and disadvantage. Others have argued that even the most radical or politically canny anti-oppressive agenda is unlikely to yield major reductions in social or economic inequality (Williams 1999: 226). Indeed, it is arguable whether even a whole generation of social care professionals trained with these issues in mind can by themselves change economic inequalities or institutional practices markedly. The human services professional might be trapped in a situation where they might think globally but have to act very locally indeed.

Thus, while individual practitioners might be aware of the difficulties facing clients, there may be little they can effectively do about many of these. The study of communication then perhaps needs to pursue a more programmatic, 'action-research' role which addresses the difficulties of communicating effectively with policymakers, media organizations and more powerful members of the communities in question so as to effectively address inequality. Whereas this would be an unusual role for communication scholars and educators to take, some clues as to its direction might be found in the work of scholars such as Prilleltensky, Preston-Shoot and Connor and colleagues. In this way we can begin to understand how the cultural field can be tilted so as to be more in favour of the voices and people who have so far been marginalized.

If we see the health care environment as a cultural field where participants, if they are to be successful, must acquire a particular kind of habitus or suite of embodied dispositions or predispositions, then the question for educators is how best to enable people to become familiar with the cultures peculiar to health care. In a sense we are dealing with a process of socialization which may be every bit as complex and far reaching as the process of being socialized into the broader culture as a whole.

Habitus, in Bourdieu's sense, refers to more than simply character, morality, or socialization *per se*, but to 'deep structural' propensities towards classification assessment, judgment, taste and understanding. These are socially acquired, and manifested in outlooks, opinions, and embodied phenomena such as deportment, posture, ways of walking, sitting, spitting, blowing the nose, and so forth as well as language itself. Habitus underlies such second-nature human characteristics and their many possible variations in different historical and cultural settings including those in health care.

Learning the language of health care

While language is not the whole of habitus, we can certainly learn a lot about what is going on in health care through the study of the language which is used there. Learning the language of health care and the kinds of problems which people bring to health care practitioners, we can learn a good deal about the essential features which are important to clients and practitioners. A careful study of health care language may well have a good deal to offer practitioners in training. By analogy with the process of acquiring a second language, there are possibilities for data-driven learning where students can explore the kinds of communication that take place in health care settings using data archives and large bodies of pre-collected data.

We would suggest that learning a new discipline such as medicine or nursing may well have much in common with learning a new language, and becoming proficient in one's chosen discipline involves new ways of thinking, talking and writing, as revealed in any comparison of novice with experienced practitioners (Crawford et al. 1999). There are perhaps opportunities for education in health care communication that might be explored in the compilation and investigation of corpora, that is bodies, databases or archives of health care-related language. This might yield important opportunities for data-driven learning in health care communication.

A data-driven learning approach would involve learners getting a 'feel' for the language of the health care encounter, by personally experiencing a focused study of the target language's organic consistencies (Johns and King 1991; Chalker 1994). In the study of language more generally there has been a good deal of interest in creating large 'corpora' of the chosen language to facilitate detailed study. So far this has been of great interest to lexicographers, linguists and sociologists of language. Rietveld et al. (2004) note that the use of corpora has become common in language research over the last few decades. In many branches of linguistics, corpora provide core data for the development and testing of hypotheses.

The concept of data-driven learning as a way of teaching was originally developed in the learning of modern languages, where, rather than learn, say, how verbs behave in different tenses, it was deemed better to enable learners to explore the language and test out their own theories about how it works. We believe that there are important lessons in data-driven learning which could productively inform the study of health language and which could enhance the education of health care practitioners. To the novice, the health care work environment may well be a kind of foreign country.

The study of corpora forms part of a number of empirical innovations in linguistics, where over the last few decades the development of large scale bodies of language has proceeded apace. The present-day interest in corpora has been described as a 'corpus revolution' (Leech 2000) such that an increasing number of scholars are concerned to develop large transcribed archives of English. This offers the opportunity to probe into the 'terra incognita' of spoken language (Carter and McCarthy 1995). Whereas conversation analysis has sometimes had the ambition to examine regular, repeatable features of interaction, it is the corpus revolution that makes this ambition possible through the availability of larger scale bodies of the spoken language.

Most famously in the UK, The Bank of English at the University of Birmingham, held as part of the COBUILD project, has in excess of 450 million words and is one of the largest collections of English language available for scholarship. The largest in the world is currently the Cambridge International Corpus, held at Cambridge University Press which comprises 1 billion words of spoken and written British and American English. At Nottingham University, where two of the present authors are based, the Cambridge and Nottingham Corpus of Discourse in English (CANCODE), begun in 1994, focuses explicitly on spoken language. Funded by Cambridge University Press as part of the Cambridge International Corpus this presently contains 5 million words of transcribed data. The recordings were collected in Britain between 1995 and 2002, keyboarded by trained transcribers, coded, and stored in a computerized database which can be searched with the publishers' specially designed software. So far the material has been used largely for projects concerning the teaching of spoken English.

Equipped with such resources and with access to powerful software packages, the present-day researcher can explore the spoken word much more readily than in the early days of linguistics. Much of the classic work in language scholarship was performed without the benefit of the quantum leap in language awareness which corpus linguistics affords.

To appreciate the applicability of this to the teaching of health care professionals, let us take a short detour into the field of language learning. Corpus linguistics perhaps offers the possibility for a more fully evidence-based approach to studying and learning about the uses of language in different settings. As Hadley (2002) argues, this has already been observed to have had a profound effect on language teaching. Indeed according to some, there has been a major paradigm shift (Woodward 1996). Starting as far back as the-mid 1980s (Swan 1985), some began to question many aspects of the way the English language was being taught to non-native speakers. This has led to an increasingly desperate search for new ways of addressing the problems encountered in language teaching. One solution, described by a number of authors, including Hadley (2002), is to make increasing use of corpora of the language being taught.

Johns and King (1991: 2) formulate the situation even more explicitly. In their work the 'language-learner is also, essentially, a research worker whose learning needs to be driven by access to linguistic data – hence the term "data-driven learning" (DDL) to describe the approach'. Data-driven learning makes explicit use of the kinds of corpora we have just been describing where learners investigate language with concordancing software. This enables learners to isolate common patterns in authentic language samples. It has been termed a new form of grammatical 'consciousness-raising' (Rutherford and Smith 1988) that attempts to move learners along the pedagogic continuum from product to process. While still very much a new methodology, DDL has been argued to be a powerful tool in teaching grammar successfully.

While it is having an impact on language teaching and learning, the possibilities for corpus research and teaching in health care have been relatively under-explored. Some of the possibilities were outlined originally by Thomas and Wilson (1996), in the case of doctor–patient interaction, but these possibilities have not so far been exploited fully.

As corpus linguistics is only just coming to be used in the study of health communication it is difficult to know yet how to evaluate it. Moreover, once we detect sociolinguistic features in health care encounters it is an even more problematic task to decide whether they are desirable and whether they are features we wish to encourage from health care professionals in the future.

The data that many authors have so far collected concerning interactions between health professionals and clients are often the result of carefully staged investigations in specific research programmes. Consequently, a wider use of more lifelike clinical encounters for teaching purposes might be advantageous. Learning the skills of the clinical encounter is a little like learning a new language. In the same way that the use of corpus linguistics has revolutionized the study of language learning and has highlighted the way that some of what is taught in conventional curricula may well be actively misleading. This is why some contemporary scholars of language learning have been so keen to advocate a data-driven learning approach. We wish to make a similar plea for health care language and health care education, so that there is an increasing role for real data in the learning and teaching of health care communication.

As Mishan (2004) notes, the many advantages of using authentic rather than purpose written materials for language learning have now been appreciated by the teaching community. Authentic texts and conversational exchanges have a richness of cultural and linguistic content which is unmatched in more artificial materials, and with a large corpus there are opportunities to select materials that are useful to specific groups of learners. There may be important motivational aspects of learning which are enhanced through the use of real as opposed to didactic material, an argument carried further by O'Keefe et al. in their aptly titled *From Corpus to Classroom* (forthcoming).

Thus there are implications here for how health care communication might be taught in future, if corpus linguistics, the study of health care language and medical teaching are brought progressively closer together. Learning a new discipline such as medicine or nursing may well have much in common with learning a new language, and becoming proficient in one's chosen discipline involves new ways of thinking, talking and writing, as revealed in any comparison of novice with experienced practitioners (Crawford et al. 1999). In the mutual exchange of a health care encounter there may be a whole variety of speech actions, which each have their own functionality. A simple question such as 'how are you?' for example may be a conversation opener or a request for a display of symptoms, depending on the context (Coupland et al. 1994).

There are a number of researchers, theorists and pedagogues in the field of language learning who stress the need to use real-life examples in the teaching of new languages. As Sinclair (1997: 30) exhorts 'present real examples only'. Widdowson (2000) highlights that this cannot form a complete pedagogy in its own right and that further understanding of the teaching and learning process may be necessary.

To provide an idea of how a corpus of language could be used in health care, we shall describe a study of our own within the Health Language Research Group at Nottingham University. It concerns a rather specific corpus that has been assembled in collaboration with the proprietors of a UK-based website containing health advice for adolescents. The site is called Teenage Health Freak (www.teenagehealthfreak.org/homepage/index.asp) and is run by Dr Ann McPherson and Dr Aidan MacFarlane. The website features an electronic equivalent of an 'agony' page such that readers are invited to send in messages with problems and selected ones will be answered on the website. The popularity of this has been very great indeed, and while only a tiny fraction of the messages are answered the number of messages written in to the website has resulted in over a million words of emails becoming available.

At the time of writing, just under half of the material available in this database of emails has been compiled into a corpus and Table 7.1 provides an indication of the most frequent words. These appear more than one would expect in the English language as a whole, based on a comparison with the CANCODE corpus.

Table 7.1   Frequencies of words in the 'teenage email' corpus

N	WORD	FREQUENCY
1	MY	9775
2	I	25,287
3	AM	3594
4	SEX	3208
5	IM	2234
6	ME	4659
7	PENIS	1480
8	HELP	1834
9	QUIZ	1273
10	ANN	1184
11	DONT	1110
12	ASKED	1443
13	PREGNANT	1092
14	QUESTION	1374
15	HAVE	6237
16	IS	6924
17	DO	5655
18	BOYFRIEND	848
19	BULLYING	785
20	PERIOD	884
21	DR	821
22	PLEASE	1265
23	DRUGS	757
24	HOW	2377
25	WORRIED	744
26	U	743
27	GAY	616
28	NORMAL	746

Note. Keywords based on a comparison of 400,000 word sub-sample of adolescent health emails and the 5 million word CANCODE corpus

It is no surprise that in the teenage email corpus first person pronouns and connected terms like 'am' are very frequently observed. What is interesting though is the sheer frequency of terms related to sexual health. Although the website solicits input across a whole range of health issues, it is sexuality and reproductive health that predominate in the emails, inasmuch as terms like 'penis', 'pregnant', 'period' and 'gay' feature far more frequently than they do in English as a whole. A few other oddities relate to the website itself. 'Ann' corresponds to the character 'Dr Ann' who acts as the agony aunt, and 'quiz' corresponds to the quizzes the website presents as a means of providing educational material – 'So you think you know about AIDS?' and so on.

The analysis of corpus material allows a process of 'drilling down' to address progressively more detailed and contextualized levels of analysis once the main features of the terrain have been apprehended. Let us take as an example the word 'normal' which appears more frequently in the present corpus than in English as a whole. Some examples of how the authors of the messages used the terms are in the box below shown below in a randomly selected concordance of 'normal':

I'm 12, I'm 5 3 ft and 42kg is this a **normal** weight or is it too light?
or being flat chested. worried boobs arent **normal** size. episodes of Bulimia and oft
seen that is normal. But i dont want to b **normal** i want to be thin. I find it insulting
14 and i havent started my period am i **normal** 8687.
sick for no apparant reason 13583. is it **normal** to miss a period for 3 months i
thinking about becoming a transexual. Is it **normal** to do this?
been a little depressed recently. Is this **normal**?
ward and i havent got any pubic hair am i **normal**? 19030. i am 13 and my name I

Here, the uses of 'normal' can be seen to relate to a variety of issues, such as mood, sex or age-related norms, such as when it is usual to begin one's periods or how regular they should be, presumably when one is in the early stages of maturity. Equally, one might say that the term normal is freighted with other meanings and positive valuations. That is, to someone concerned about weight or height, normal might connote an imagined normative notion of health, whereas to someone concerned about the onset of periods the normativity might refer to the desirability of not being left out when one's peers begin menstruating. If we take a more fully developed picture of the contexts in which normal occurred it is more obvious what it is doing in the correspondents' questions. A selection of questions from the teenage health corpus including the word 'normal' is presented in the box below.

I am addicted to cerial. Is this **normal**?

hi only one of my balls have droped, is this **normal**? will the other one drop in time?

Hi dr A. i fink iv started my periods but im not sure coz it woz brown. i told my mum and she sed i had started and it was **normal** 4 my fist period. but im stil worried coz sumtimes ders brown stuf and sumtimes ders nowt der. plz help?

when i smoke the smoke comes out of my ears sometimes

i want to know if this is **normal** they can also be painfull when i go swimming or my head goes underwater

i don't look fat but i have a small bit of flab on my stomach that doesn't look very nice and would put be of wearing anything

that doesn't cover it. i weigh 9 stone is that **normal**? i am 165 cm tall! sometimes i will diet my self for 2 weeks and i will go down to 8 and a half stone but in one week put it all back on! should i be on a permenat diet?

is enlarged pupils **normal**?

Is it **normal** to have peeling skin on my hands?

Looking at the way normality and its opposites are formulated in these questions it appears that it is often part of a contrastive statement, such that the event or phenomenon is described and then an invited contrast or comparison is posed, 'is this normal?' It may not be speculating too much to see the term 'normal' as one which indicates stance (Precht 2003) and appraisal (Macken-Horarik 2003). That is, when people say 'normal' in this corpus it is often in the context of something they think is wrong, rather than in the sense of being merely curious as to whether things are statistically usual.

There were also a small number of instances of the word 'normal' which were rather more difficult to interpret. Some of these atypical uses of the term 'normal' in the teenage health corpus are presented in the box below.

i am pregnant is this **normal** for a boy

i have three testicles is this **normal**

i am 3 and i have started my period is this **normal**

I'm a transexual, is it **normal**?

There are various ways of trying to make sense of these. Maybe they are intended humorously – as if the writers had thought of things that seemed to them the most bizarre, humorous or taboo and added the question 'am I normal?' as a sort of self-referential parody. It may be of course that they are true – in which case the 3-year-old is just as advanced in her literacy skills as she is with the start of her periods.

Databases such as we are collecting can be used for the investigation of all kinds of other issues in the language. Let us take another example of a relatively high frequency term in Table 7.1, 'worried'. An examination of the corpus tells us what sorts of things people claim to be worried about. A small selection of the kinds of problems yielding usage of the term worried is presented in the box below.

- I am **worried** I may be pregnant but am still having normal regular menstrual cycles. I have taken a couple of home pregnancy tests and they say negative but Im **worried** about the time I do the tests as they say you should take it on the first day of your missed period, so if Im still having my periods, whens the best time to take the test?
- I started my period roughly two years ago. It's been quite regular, but all of a sudden, I've missed about 4 periods and still haven't come on. I've never had sex though! I'm really **worried**. Why is this and what do I do?
- dear docter Ann i have been bullied before and sorted it out, but i am **worried** it will start again after the easter term. I am also **worried** about my friend as she got bullied by a different person and had to walk home and i am **worried** if she walks home again she might get in to some situation like with a man and get kidnapped. please tell me if i am being to much of a worry wart, thankyou
- i really want to snog my boyfriend. Problem is, ihave never done it before and im not sure how! I'm **worried** i will go wrong or do the wrong thing. please help

Many of the correspondents seemed to be experiencing worry where the possibility of pregnancy or menstrual disruption were concerned. It is as if underlying this there is a substantive expectation that the cycle will be regular and departure from this occasions concern. Of course many people experience irregularity and later in life this may not be identified as a problem but in one's early experiences of menstruation regularity may be perceived as normative. Equally, worry may involve the possible negative eventualities of social situations at school or the perennial fears of being maladroit at kissing. This highlights another use of corpora such as this in exploring lay theories and folk beliefs about health and about likely eventualities in social etiquette.

Recent work by other scholars on everyday explanations for illness has disclosed a rich variety of lay explanatory frameworks. In a study by Popay et al. (2003: 7–9) explanations for ill health ranged from 'beer fags egg and chips' to 'worry and stress' and included 'worse housing, high unemployment and a lack of hope in the area'.

There may also be findings from corpus work that help us understand the relationship between language concerning health or bodily issues and how this has infused the language as a whole. Mishan (2004) reports some investigations of the occurrence of terms for body parts, averaged from the results of searches on two online corpora, namely the COBUILD Bank of English website (http://www.cobuild.collins.co.uk) and the British National Corpus online (http://sara.natcorp.ox.ac.uk). Here, for example approximately 45 per cent of the occurrences of the word 'hand' were idiomatic ('on the one hand', 'give a big hand to', 'out of hand', 'to hand', etc.). Work on idioms and idiomatic usage in health care can therefore usefully be based on the evidence of corpus research. Indeed, to anyone working in health with young people in the medium of English there could be valuable lessons to be learned. Of course, the material here does not necessarily tell us how American or Australasian teenagers would talk about the issues, nor does the data-collection process allow the questions and problems to be traced to particular class, ethnic or faith subgroups. This would have to wait upon the creation of corpora where researchers have proactively collected demographic and contextual information to accompany the language itself.

However, this highlights the role of corpus-based learning activities which can be deployed in getting students to understand the issues in health care encounters. Data-driven learning (DDL) encourages learners to engage with the corpus via research tasks, and is significant in that it is a pedagogical application of a research method, originating with Tim Johns's famous contention that 'research is too serious to be left to the researchers' (Johns and King 1991: 2). As Mishan (2004) describes it, the key feature of the methodology is this 'aura' of research, and this research agenda is what gives the sense of authenticity. In the initial work with this data we have done with health psychologists in training, nurses and counsellors there is generally a fascination with the data and a tendency to ask questions like 'How did they . . .?', 'Did anybody say . . .?' and 'Were there very many . . .?' which are, of course empirical questions which they can then go on to investigate with the data themselves. The correspondence between the kinds of questions asked by the users of the website and the air of the ever popular problem page features of magazines gives a sense of authenticity and the research element confers a sense of the genuine discoveries which still remain to be made concerning the use of language in health care.

Despite this enthusiasm for the use of authentic examples and material from corpora in teaching about health care communication, it is important to note that there are some important differences between the material included in a corpus of language and the original. 'The texts which are collected in a corpus have only a reflected reality' (Widdowson 2000: 7), for 'Reality . . . does not travel with the text' (Widdowson 1998: 711–12). The reality, the authenticity, of text is tarnished by transposition (Mishan 2004). In addition, as we have noted, there are some research questions which it would be very difficult to address in this way without considerable further research to ascertain the demographic characteristics of the correspondents.

Yet as we have argued, a data-driven learning approach might have a great deal to offer an increasingly beleaguered National Health Service in the UK. Understanding the idiomatic expressions which people in the UK (and elsewhere) use to describe their health problems, grasping the lay theories and folkways they use to interpret what has gone wrong and getting a grip on the rhythms of complaint might well be facilitated by the use of corpora of health care language. In the UK it is becoming increasingly urgent to come up with new ways of educating and training health service personnel, especially in the light of changes in the NHS workforce and rapid demographic, epidemiological and linguistic changes in the population. There seems to be little support for non-native speakers of English in the NHS, despite the large number of such employees in the organization. For example, it is estimated that 25 per cent of doctors do not have English as a first language. At present the situation is addressed by means of an examination in English, yet this is only a single-point measure, and is only applied to speakers of non-EU foreign languages.

As corpus research discloses, there is considerably more to health concerns and health care practice than simply being able to translate from one language to another and having the relevant professional qualifications. If we take the view that language is transactional, it is important to consider how the language of a health care encounter can be 'recipient tailored' (Brown and Fraser 1979). Indeed, it may well be that clients give different accounts of themselves in response to different health care professionals, even if the latter are following more or less the same assessment script.

It is particularly important to examine the issue of health language closely via corpus-based research at present because there are some important changes afoot in the health communication field. For example, the emphasis that we have already noted on working with clients and taking their views into account has gained favour with policymakers. It is through careful attention to the language of health care encounters that we will be able to document the shift from older models of information giving to more contemporarily modish approaches to 'working with the client' and suggest how it might best be expedited.

Although linguists have in the past been the main users of corpora, they certainly need not be the sole users in the future. Health scientists will increasingly require access to *naturalistic* data which cannot be reproduced in laboratory conditions, while at the same time they are under pressure to quantify and test their theories rather than rely on qualitative data.

One important topic of enquiry that is germane to this kind of study of health care relates to the kinds of explanations people give for events. The question of how and why people explain phenomena is of interest from the point of view of health psychology and health promotion. Explanations (or *attributions*) have been important to psychologists because they reveal the ways in which people regard their environment. One early corpus linguistic study of explanations by Antaki and Naji (1987) showed that explanations of general states of affairs were the most common type of explanation (33.8 per cent) followed by actions of speaker and speaker's group (28.8 per cent) and actions of others (17.7 per cent). This challenged previous social-psychological theories that the prototypical explanation is the explanation of a person's actions. Looking at how people explain things has important implications for devising educational or information-giving strategies.

In the same way, our adolescent health corpus can reveal how the correspondents conceptualize the causal relationships involved in anatomy and physiology work, as well as the operation of the social world around them. Some examples of usage of 'because' in the teenage health corpus are provided in the box below.

---

im 15 and started my periods at 12 but my tits r 34B but my hips r staright up and down and i feel like an idiot and dont like going out anymore (but i dont go out much anyway **because** of panic attacks) how can i get woman hips?

I'm am 15 and 5ft 4 inches tall. I look different to all the other girls my age **because** I'm so skinny -

if people bully you **because** you do not smoke what do you do

i dont have many friends **because** im different

please can I have sum information on losing weight I am really depressed **because** I am over weight

---

As we can see even from this small selection, there are a number of implied causal relationships that the correspondents have identified. One may be depressed 'because' of being overweight, and relationships with peers may be problematic 'because' of differences, either unspecified ones or something specific such as smoking. Equally, personal theories about the relationship between staying in and the likelihood of panic attacks are implicated in the loops of causal relationships too, as are the consequences of being 'skinny'. This then provides a resource for understanding what the term 'because' is used for and by implication how causal relationships are conceptualized.

We would therefore argue that progress in the health care disciplines may best be served by taking a leaf out of the modern linguists' book and using a similar approach to deal with teaching and learning health care language. Moreover, it might well be possible to link communicative styles, strategies and motifs to data concerning the effectiveness of health care interventions. In this way a more effective and evidence-based approach to health care language can be developed which will promote the best use of class time for trainees and scarce and expensive resources such as drugs and treatment facilities.

Conclusion: learning lessons

In this chapter we have attempted to highlight some new trends and possibilities in the learning of health care communication skills which have some promise to shift the envelope of debate about health care communication and the way in which it can be taught.

We began with some theories about learning and pedagogy which highlight the way that so much of what is studied as learning and teaching has tended to concentrate on what the learner does and what he or she knows. From there we moved on to consider some more socialized understandings of the teaching and learning process and the acquisition of expertise. Here, the work of Freire and Bourdieu is relevant as well as the role of informal learning and communities of practice passing on their accumulated social capital. We also considered some of the attempts to theorize power and social context in the lives of practitioners and clients, via notions of empowerment and anti-oppressive practice. Relating this back to our main theme of the evidence base of communication, these issues of course do not necessarily add to the stock of evidence in themselves yet they help us towards a more critical appreciation of the evidence itself. It assists us in making sense of the assumptions made by overly individualistic accounts of the acquisition of communication skills. It also allows us to determine whose interests are served by particular research enterprises, communication advice or political perspectives.

Finally, our account of corpus-based and data-driven learning in health care has shown how new ways of making sense of language have a place in the education of health care practitioners. Whereas these kinds of ideas will probably never replace the sorts of education for health professionals which we saw in the previous chapter, it is appropriate to show how these techniques can extend the work of educators and raise the consciousness of practitioners. It is unique in that it can show a great deal of the texture and feel of health care communication and convey some of the richness of everyday communication about health care issues. It is this feature which makes it important as an educational resource and which will enable these kinds of approaches to add value over and above what is achievable with selected and staged material that might be used in role-plays or hypothetical examples.

References

Abbott, E., Abbott, G. and Firestone, S. (1997) *Women's Issues*, Vol. 1. Pasadena, CA: Salem Press.

Antaki, C. and Naji, S. (1987) Events explained in conversational 'because' statements, *British Journal of Social Psychology*, 26: 119–26.

Biggs, J. (1999) *Teaching for Quality Learning at University: What the Student Does*. Buckingham: Society for Research into Higher Education and Open University Press.

Bloom, B. (1956) *Taxonomy of Educational Objectives, Handbook I: Cognitive Domain*. New York: Longman.

Bourdieu, P. (1984) *Distinction: A Social Critique of the Judgment of Taste*. Cambridge, MA: Harvard University Press.

Bourdieu, P. (1986) The forms of capital, in J.G. Richardson (ed.) *Handbook of Theory and Research for the Sociology of Education*. New York: Greenwood Press.

Bourdieu, P. (1991) *Language and Symbolic Power*. Cambridge, MA: Harvard University Press.

Bourdieu, P. (1998) *Practical Reason*. Palo Alto, CA: Stanford University Press.

Bransford, J.D., Brown, A.L. and Cocking, R.R. (1999) *How People Learn: Brain, Mind Experience and School*. Washington, DC: National Academy Press.

Brown, P. and Fraser, C. (1979) Speech as a marker of situation, in K.R. Scherer and H. Giles (eds) *Social Markers in Speech*. Cambridge: Cambridge University Press.

Carter, R. and McCarthy, M. (1995) Grammar and the spoken language, *Applied Linguistics*, 16(2): 141–58.

Chalker, S. (1994) Pedagogical grammar: principles and problems, in M. Bygate, A. Tonkyn and E. Williams (eds) *Grammar and the Language Teacher*. London: Prentice Hall.

Connor, A., Ling, C.G., Tuttle, J. and Brown-Tezera, B. (1999) Peer education project with persons who have experienced homelessness, *Public Health Nursing*, 16(5): 367–73.

Coupland, J., Robinson, J.D. and Coupland, N. (1994) Frame negotiation in doctor–elderly patient interactions, *Discourse and Society*, 5: 89–124.

Crawford, P., Johnson, A.J., Brown, B. and Nolan, P. (1999) The language of mental health nursing reports: firing paper bullets? *Journal of Advanced Nursing*, 29(2): 331–40.

Curr, D. (1994) Role play, *British Medical Journal*, 308: 725.

Custers, E.J.F.M. and Boshuizen, H.P.A. (2002) The psychology of learning, in G.R. Norman, C.P.M. Van Der Vleuten and D.I. Newble (eds) *International Handbook of Research in Medical Education*. Dordrecht: Kluwer.

D'Eon, M. (2004) A blueprint for inter-professional learning, *Medical Teacher*, 26(7): 604–9.

Dewar, B.J. and Walker, E. (1999) Experiential learning: issues for supervision, *Journal of Advanced Nursing*, 30(6): 1459–67.

Dunphy, B.C. and Williamson, S.L. (2004) In pursuit of expertise: toward an educational model for expertise development, *Advances in Health Sciences Education*, 9: 107–27.

Eraut, M. (1994) *Developing Professional Knowledge and Competence*. London: Falmer Press.

Hadley, G. (2002) Sensing the winds of change: an introduction to data-driven learning, *RELC Journal*, 33(2): 99–124.

Hart, A., Hall, V. and Henwood, F. (2003) Helping health and social care professionals to develop an 'inequalities imagination': a model for use in education and practice, *Journal of Advanced Nursing*, 41(5): 480–9.

Johns, T.F. and King, P. (1991) *Classroom Concordancing*. Birmingham: ELR.

Lave, J. and Wenger, E. (1991) *Situated Learning: Legitimate Peripheral Participation*. Cambridge: Cambridge University Press.

Leech, G. (2000) Grammars of spoken English: new outcomes of corpus oriented research, *Language Learning*, 50(4): 675–724.

Lindwall, L., von Post, I. and Bergbom, I. (2003) Patients' and nurses' experience of perioperative dialogues, *Journal of Advanced Nursing*, 43(3): 246–53.

Macken-Horarik, M. (2003) Appraisal and the special instructiveness of narrative, *Text*, 23(2): 285–312.

Mackway-Jones, K. and Walker, M. (1999) *The Pocket Guide to Teaching for Medical Instructors*. London: BMJ Books.

Miller, J.F. (1992) *Coping with Chronic Illness: Overcoming Powerlessness*, 2nd edn. Philadelphia, PA: F.A. Davis Company.

Mishan, F. (2004) Authenticating corpora for language learning: a problem and its resolution, *ELT Journal*, 58(3): 219–27.

O'Keeffe, A., McCarthy, M., and Carter, R. (forthcoming) *From Corpus to Classroom: Grammar, Vocabulary and Discourse. Cambridge: Cambridge University Press.*

O'Keeffe, M., White, D., Spurrier, N. and Fox, N. (2001) An inter-university community child health clinical placement programme for medical students, *Medical Education*, 35(4): 384–90.

Patvardhan, C. (2005) Tips on breaking bad news, *British Medical Journal*, 330: 1131.

Popay, J., Bennett, S., Thomas, C., Williams, G., Gatrell, A. and Bostock, L. (2003) Beyond 'beer, fags, egg and chips'? Exploring lay understandings of social inequalities in health, *Sociology of Health and Illness*, 25(1): 1–23.

Pratt, D.D. (1998) *Five Perspectives on Teaching in Adult and Higher Education*. Malabar, FL: Krieger Publishing Company.

Precht, K. (2003) Stance moods in spoken English: evidentiality and affect in British and American conversation, *Text*, 23(2): 239–57.

Preston-Shoot, M. (1995) Assessing anti-oppressive practice, *Social Work Education*, 14: 11–29.

Prilleltensky, I. (2005) Promoting well-being: time for a paradigm shift in health and human services, *Scandinavian Journal of Public Health*, 33 (Suppl. 66): 53–60.

Rietveld, T., Van Hout, R. and Ernestus, M. (2004) Pitfalls in corpus research, *Computers and the Humanities*, 38: 343–62.

Rutherford, W. and Smith, M. (1988) Consciousness raising and universal grammar, in W. Rutherford and M. Smith (eds) *Grammar and Second Language Teacher: A Book of Readings*. Boston: Heinle and Heinle.

Salomon, G. (ed.) (1993) *Distributed Cognition: Psychological and Educational Considerations*. Cambridge: Cambridge University Press.

Shipengrover, J.A. and James, P.A. (1999) Measuring instructional quality in community-orientated medical education: looking into the black box, *Medical Education*, 33: 846–53.

Sinclair, J.M. (1997) Corpus evidence in language description, in A. Wichman and S. Fligelstone (eds.) *Teaching and Language Corpora*. London: Longman.

Swan, M. (1985) A critical look at the communicative approach, *ELT Journal*, 39(1): 2–12.

Thomas, J. and Wilson, A. (1996) Methodologies for studying a corpus of doctor–patient interaction, in J. Thomas and M. Short, (eds) *Using Corpora for Language Research*. London: Longman.

Wallerstein, N. (1992) Powerlessness, empowerment, and health: Implications for health promotion programs, *American Journal of Health Promotion*, 6(3): 197–205.

Widdowson, H.G. (1998) Context, community and authentic language, *TESOL Quarterly*, 32(4): 705–16.

Widdowson, H.G. (2000) On the limitations of linguistics applied, *Applied Linguistics*, 21(1): 3–25.

Williams, C. (1999) Connecting anti-racist and anti-oppressive theory and practice: retrenchment or reappraisal? *British Journal of Social Work*, 29: 211–30.

Wilkinson, T.J., Gower, S. and Sainsbury, R. (2002) The earlier, the better: the effect of early community contact on the attitudes of medical students to older people, *Medical Education*, 36(6): 540–2.

Woodward, T. (1996) Paradigm shift and the language teaching profession, in J. Willis and D. Willis (eds) *Challenge and Change in Language Teaching*. Oxford: Heinemann.

8 Communicating carefully: communicating about sensitive matters

Care and communication

In this chapter we will examine the special circumstances where communications are undertaken around issues which are sensitive, emotive or taboo. Matters relating to sexuality, terminal illness, possible illegal activities or even spiritual beliefs all come under the rubric of health care, and professionals and clients regularly communicate about them. However, unlike describing the common cold or a bad back there are often distinctive features to the kind of communication undertaken about 'delicate matters'.

For example, there may be a kind of baby talk deployed in the context of gynaecological consultations, or a euphemistic vocabulary in continence care. In this chapter we will attempt to map out what has been researched on these topics and describe the functions of these different styles of communication. From the practitioner's point of view, novice health professionals are often apprehensive about approaching these issues with clients and we will distil from the literature examples of how effective communication might be achieved most appropriately. In dealing with different ethnic groups and different languages there may be particular difficulties. For example, the highly specific terminology of HIV medicine and counselling needs special attention. Many bilingual practitioners get their HIV training in English, and then are at a loss on how to translate words such as 'risk reduction' and 'viral load'. Especially in the case of contentious or delicate matters, there is increasing evidence that language plays a critical role in increasing access, improving quality, and reducing health care disparities for the diverse people health professionals serve in communities across the globe.

Sexuality, sexual health and communicating with care

One of the major areas where sensitivity is demanded is that of sexual and reproductive health. As Serrant-Green (2005) reminds us, this area has through much of human history been associated with social taboo, shame, secrecy and blame. The picture of sexual health has undergone some rapid shifts in the last 20 years or so with concerns about HIV and AIDS. Yet long before the discovery of HIV and AIDS, sexual activity in many cultures had been infused by fears and concerns about immorality and in the West at least by medical and sexological notions about what was 'normal' as well as fears about moral decline.

Sexual health, despite the investment of resources and effort over the last 20 years has thus had a Cinderella status, with many researchers and practitioners seeing it as a soft option or 'not real medicine'. Sexuality and to some extent reproductive issues over the years have existed under a veil of silence that has been difficult to overcome. In popular culture, of course, sexuality has flourished and forms the basis of thriving industries as well as a progressive sexualization of mainstream entertainment. Yet knowledge about sexual difficulties, even if it appears to be medically sanctioned, is often partial and difficult for people to apply in their own case, and when advice fails to work people are often inclined to blame themselves rather than the advice givers, and worry that they are not 'normal', as we have seen in the previous chapter.

The privatization of sex and genitourinary anatomy has not always been a feature of the western cultural landscape. A good deal of the privacy, furtiveness and shame surrounding this was constructed in the seventeenth and eighteenth centuries (Laqueur 2003). There is thus a distinctive 'habitus' or speech genre concerned with talking about sexual, reproductive or genitourinary health which repays scrutiny as this tells us a great deal about how communicative practices relate to broader social values, norms and taboos.

In thinking about the pattern of speech and writing about sexuality and reproductive health, making sense of the 'genre' of speech in that context might be desirable (Trinch 2001). A genre is a 'class' or 'kind' of text, and is frequently used as a way of classifying and describing films, such as westerns, musicals and so on. The idea of genres has aroused some controversy, but many contemporary theorists tend to describe genres in terms of 'family resemblances' among texts, rather than obeying a single strict definition (Swales 1990: 49). An individual text, film or clinical discourse will rarely if ever have all of the characteristic features of the genre to which it belongs (Fowler 1989: 215). Thus, while it is not straightforward to talk about a 'genre' of clinical conversations about sexual or reproductive health, for the moment let us pursue the idea because it brings with it some powerful concepts that will help us crack open what is going on in such situations. One early twentieth century theorist who tried to use the concept of genres to characterize language and communicative activity was Mikhail Bakhtin (1986: 60), according to whom any particular speech genre can be seen as the product of a specific 'sphere of communication' and that speech genres 'reflect the specific conditions and goals' of their sites of production and reception.

These goals are manifested 'through [the genre's] thematic content, the selection of the lexical, phraseological, and grammatical resources of the language, and above all through compositional structure' (Bakhtin 1986: 60). By now the reader should already be familiar with the view of many sociolinguists who would consider any conversation or speech act to be an emergent product of the joint efforts of the parties present and participating in the making of the discourse (Schiffrin 1994; Ewick and Silbey 1995). Combining Bakhtin's notion of speech genres with a sociolinguistic approach to the study of narrative in professional contexts (Bhatia 1993) provides a useful starting point from which to investigate contexts of construction that inform discussions of reproductive and sexual health. Generally, researchers interested in the nature of human sexual decision making, for example, are hindered by the fact that the subject, the practices and the parts of the body involved are still perceived as being 'not nice', too sensitive for 'objective' research or unlikely to provide truthful responses in research data (Pitts 1996).

This relationship between genre and context is illustrated in a study by Stewart (2005) of the hygiene practices adopted by midwives in examining their clients going through childbirth. As Stewart notes, women's bodies have been viewed as problematic in many historical and cultural contexts and seen as a potential source of dirt and pollution. She notes that perhaps vaginal examinations during labour might be used as a ritual procedure by which health care professionals demonstrate their control of the labouring woman and the labour process itself.

It has often been noted by researchers that health care professionals use rituals to make care of the body and its 'dirty work' socially manageable (Lawler 1991; Bergstrom et al. 1992; Twigg 2000). The meticulous procedure adopted in such cases by some midwives can be seen as a ritual to help deal with their own discomfort at performing something so intimate. Yet perhaps, as Stewart (2005) suggests, the procedure is more than a means of dealing with embarrassment, and these sometimes highly ritualized washing procedures can also imply a display of professional power and constitute part of a disciplinary regime aimed at containing women's 'leaky' bodies within a stable and controllable framework (Shildrick 1997: 11).

In Stewart's (2005) study also, there was in some cases an apparent reluctance to talk about the process of performing a vaginal examination or washing the area in question. Euphemisms and abbreviations were used instead – 'an internal' or a 'VE' instead of 'vaginal examination'. This process has sometimes been called 'verbal asepsis', and has been seen as an aspect of the power strategies whereby midwives decide what information will be given to women and what will be withheld. Equally, in Stewart's study, midwives also use these abbreviations as a form of 'verbal asepsis' in discussion with professional peers and the interviewer, and in situations outside the clinical arena.

Thus it is as if there is a distinctive genre of clinical talk and related clinical practice where the genitourinary system is concerned. As well as Stewart's (2005) study, there are others where similar kinds of circumlocution are apparent. One way is to infantilize the client with terms of endearment – as the title of Bergstrom et al.'s (1992) article has it: 'You'll feel me touching you sweetie'.

This kind of circumlocution or elliptical talk can be observed in some textbooks too. For example, while the physical practicalities of vaginal examination might be discussed, there is little corresponding discussion of how the procedure can be discussed with clients. As one textbook says of vaginal examination, it 'is an essential skill for the midwife ... [and] should be undertaken sensitively due to the intimate nature of the examination' (Johnson and Taylor: 179). The authors describe the procedure in detail but, apart from stating that the midwife should 'gain informed consent and ensure privacy' (p. 183), no further advice is given as to the communicative strategy which might best be adopted. Over 30 years ago, one account of vaginal examinations in the context of gynaecological assessment suggested that doctors must attempt to treat a woman 'as an object with their hands' but at the same time 'as a person with their voices' (Emerson 1971).

The pattern we have noted above where it appears that there is relatively little effective communication surrounding birth and genitourinary medicine and that parts of the body and procedures are shrouded in silence, is repeated across a number of other studies. In an account of patients who had sustained perineal damage in childbirth, Williams et al. (2005) note that there were a number of aspects of the communicative experience that participants found problematic. For example, even when information was provided, it was sometimes communicated in a very rushed way:

> Well, all the midwives seemed, they just seemed so busy, it's just as if they need to double up the amount of staff because they were just so busy and they haven't really got time to sit with you and discuss things, and I just think there was a serious lack of communication. (FG1, participant 1)

(p. 131)

Participants reported feeling their expectations were often unfulfilled in terms of their questions being answered by practitioners.

> With everyone I asked – midwives, doctors – it was almost like they don't want to commit themselves to facts or, you know, all very vague. I was wanting information and help, and no one ever really seemed to know. (FG2, participant 2)

(p. 132)

Now from the practitioners' point of view there may be considerable uncertainty – it is often difficult to predict how a wound will heal and the degree of pain and functional impairment the client will undergo, and how long it might last. Yet clients are desperate for information in a situation with many uncertainties. Yet once again we see the signs of a speech genre which is specific to obstetric, gynaecological and genitourinary settings, where communication is conspicuous by its absence. Perhaps the taboos surrounding those parts of the body, the reticence of the staff, who are often relatively young and recently out of training themselves, the awkwardness that patients might feel, despite their curiosity to know what is happening to them, all conspire to sustain the silence.

The memories of childbirth can cause feelings of misunderstanding, guilt, anger and confusion, which are connected with anxiety, depression, and even reluctance to consider future pregnancies (Lavender and Walkinshaw 1998). Loss of control, physical pain, emotional and sexual difficulties, and lack of information were sources of anxiety after childbirth of any form, no matter whether there was any tissue damage (Glazener 1997).

In relation to the communication needs surrounding perineal damage in childbirth, Williams et al. (2005) argue that the timing and amount of information given to women is important. This obstetric complication occurs amidst an event which is already emotionally demanding, with a number of other feelings over new motherhood and concern for the infant which may conflict with the need to come to terms with the injuries sustained. Williams and colleagues believe it is important for women with perineal injuries to be adequately informed, such that all the staff are aware of the recommended practice for repair of these injuries, so they can answer questions and explain what is happening (Thakar and Sultan 2003). Williams et al. (2005) also recommend a dedicated team for the counselling and follow-up of women suffering these injuries, with continuity of care and establishment of a degree of trust, as well as actively involving the women's partners so that they are able to offer emotional support, and address their own anxieties. In a sense then, Williams and colleagues are advocating a change at the level of culture and speech genre concerning perineal health following childbirth. The present situation is reminiscent of what Grossen and Apotheloz (1998) and Allan and Burridge (1991) described when they examined the use of euphemism, circumlocution, or even not mentioning things at all, as strategies speakers use to avoid face-threatening acts (Brown and Levinson 1987) when talking about sensitive, delicate or culturally inappropriate conversational topics. The diffi-culty then is to ensure that participants' needs for information are met yet their dignity is attended to.

One example of a study suggesting that professionals had achieved a suitable balance comes from a study of a nurse-led continence service by Shaw et al. (2000) which yielded some clues as to the kind of attitude and demeanour that is valued in such circumstances. For example 'friendly' was the most frequently occurring positive adjective used by clients to describe good experiences with the nurses:

I: What do you find makes a good service?

R: Well, it depends a lot on the person you are dealing with, and C— made it easy. She is the sort of person that, well she is ideal for that sort of thing. She is so friendly, so open and you can talk to her about anything. It was good. (Id 18 Female)

(p. 576)

Thus as this quote suggests, 'good communication' was closely related to the sense of being 'friendly'. Equally, where personal disclosures were reciprocal, and the con-versation ranged beyond purely professional matters, patients appreciated this and were more likely to divulge information when the relationship had some degree of informality: clients felt that the friendliness resulted in mutual respect and a sense of equality that they found empowering.

These kinds of initiatives where the friendliness and approachability of the per-sonnel are foregrounded seem to represent a popular and effective way of ensuring that clients are satisfied and engage productively with services. Indeed, like the advice in the earlier chapters, much of this seems so straightforward as to be facile. As John Skelton, a prominent UK health communication educator has remarked, surely no one would advise practitioners to be rude, brusque or off-putting.

Nevertheless, the fear that health professionals will react this way to enquiries about sexual health appears still to be widespread especially among youngsters. The British Medical Association (2005) reports a recent survey of young people conducted in conjunction with the charity Developing Patient Partnerships which suggested that youngsters would be reticent about asking for advice. Forty-six per cent of 16–24-year-olds who took part in the survey said that they would find it embarrassing to discuss sexual health with a GP or nurse. Forty-five per cent mistakenly thought that they had to see their GP before they could access sexual health services, despite the willingness of many genitourinary medicine facilities in the UK to see self-referred patients. In the same survey 82 per cent said that more information on what to expect from a visit to a sexual health clinic or GP surgery would make it more likely that they would get the help they needed. In line with the principles of open access which operate in the UK's genitourinary medicine and many 'drop in' or 'walk in' facilities 67 per cent said they would prefer to remain anonymous when trying to get help and information. Perhaps connected with this desire for anonymity 78 per cent cited online information as the preferred source of help.

It is perhaps difficult to reconcile the desirability of an informal and friendly approach to sensitive matters which was noted to be successful earlier, and the impersonality which is being demanded by many young people. It is important to note that while the evidence reported here may usefully inform strategies of communication, we are far from achieving knowledge of any universal truths about communication in sensitive contexts.

Diversity: room for improvement?

In considering ethnic diversity, the first sensitive matter is how to define or classify the diverse range of ethnic and cultural groups involved. There are a number of aspects which researchers and census enumerators have identified, all of which have well-known shortcomings. We might try to identify the ethnic group from which a person comes in terms of country of origin, self-identified ethnic status, language spoken, the religion they practise, or where their family originated. Whatever index is taken, there are complications and exceptions. Identifying ethnic groups by means of biological markers is complicated by the similarity between human groups compared with the diversity within them and by the fact that very few human populations have ever lived in complete isolation. Equally, there is a disturbingly close relationship sometimes encountered between broad ethnic classifications and theorists claiming that ethnic differences in health, achievement, income or offending behaviour are somehow constitutional in origin.

Despite these difficulties, it is clear from examination of any major centre of population in the UK that Britain has long been a country of migration (Parekh 2000) and that patterns of different groups' and nationalities' migration to Britain have a varied history. Since World War II, and until recently, immigration to the UK was dominated by people from countries which were formerly connected with the British Empire, especially South Asia, the Caribbean and Africa. In the mid years of the twentieth century, immigration was predominantly from the Caribbean and India. Later, in the 1960s and 1970s more migrants arrived in the UK from India and Pakistan, and people from East Africa who were of Asian ancestry. Migrants from Bangladesh arrived during the 1980s. As Alexander et al. (2004) note, recently the picture has shifted once again and refugee and asylum claims from populations in Africa, the Middle East and Eastern Europe have been a feature (see also Dustmann et al. 2003).

The issue of migration and ethnic grouping is particularly fraught because in many parts of the world it is associated with inequality and discrimination. Racism itself may have profound health consequences (Karlsen and Nazroo 2002), yet these have been under-researched. The experience of racism can have direct physical consequences, and can become internalized, damaging self-esteem, and potentially compromising the sufferer's or the community's ability to mobilize social support, which will also have consequences for health (Krieger and Sidney 1996).

Manifestly, ethnic minorities differ in culture. Culture can be broadly defined as a common heritage involving sets of beliefs, norms and values (US Department of Health and Human Services 1999). It relates to the learned attributes of groups of people. A person's 'cultural identity' may be taken to mean the culture with which they identify and to which they look for support and guidance on standards of behaviour (Cooper and Denner 1998). Culture in turn influences many variables important to health such as attitudes, diet, exercise, uses of alternative medical care, exposure to violence, family structure and many other factors. Migrants may arrive in a new country with their own culture, but may tend through acculturation and socialization to adapt over time to the dominant culture within which they live. Culture is dynamic and continually changes, under the influence of demands of the environment, politics, and strategic interventions by dominant interests. A majority culture in any country is clearly influenced by interactions with minority groups. Immigrant groups may band together and form their own culture, which may include valued aspects of the old country, but which is modified by demands of the new land (Zhou and Bankston 1998).

This dynamic process means that culture is difficult to fix and define; yet clearly there are still important inequalities and difficulties of communication in health care. As sociologist Thomas LaVeist (1996: 26) summarized, 'Race is a poor indicator of biology, a better indicator of ethnicity (culturally determined health and illness behavior) and a very good indicator of exposure to socio-environmental factors such as racism'.

In both the USA and the UK there is a long history of racial and ethnic health disparities and significant biases and inequalities in the delivery of health care. This was documented for example in a recent study by the Institute of Medicine (Smedley et al. 2003: 123) which argues that these inequalities 'occur in the context of broader historic and contemporary social and economic inequality, and are evidence of persistent racial and ethnic discrimination in many sectors of American life'. This includes the health care system itself and has important implications for how we understand communicative processes in health care settings. Ethnic minorities often find themselves in ethnic-discordant relationships with health professionals who often tend to be of the majority culture. Thus they rate both the quality of interpersonal care by practitioners, and by the health care system as a whole more negatively than whites (Cooper and Roter 2003).

Equally, researchers have regularly detected bias and stereotyping among health care providers themselves (Schulman et al. 1999; van Ryn and Burke 2000). Indeed, the cultural orientation of the medical care system is believed to be less aligned with the cultural and spiritual perspective of some patient groups than others (Taylor 2003; Wear 2003). Given the important role that interpersonal processes, including manifestations of bias and cultural competence, may play in the provision of health care to ethnic minorities (van Ryn and Fu 2003; Wear 2003), investigations of these phenomena might be important indicators of the cultural competence of individual practitioners and of the health care system as a whole.

As Johnson et al. (2004) identified in their research, African Americans were likely to believe they had been treated unfairly and with disrespect in the health care system based on the way they spoke English. This supports the suspicion that cultural differences between African Americans and their predominantly white physicians are behind this perception, even though they nominally speak the same language. Johnson et al. (2004: 108) argue that many minority groups in the USA such as Hispanics and Asians, as well as African Americans, 'are given a message that aspects of their culture, including the way they speak English, are not looked upon favourably in the health care system'.

The picture of health in developed nations is also one where ethnic, cultural and spiritual differences intersect with economic ones. For example, families from ethnic minority backgrounds in the UK are also disproportionately likely to be poor (Alexander et al. 2004; Preston 2005). In the light of these cultural, linguistic and economic differences, Campinah-Bacote's (1999) work on cultural competence is relevant. She suggests that the process of cultural competence in the delivery of health care services should be one of constant striving towards culturally competent adequate services, rather than assuming that an adequate recognition of diversity has ever been achieved. Campinah-Bacote's model involves a number of aspects, including cultural awareness, which involve appreciation of, and sensitivity to, the values and beliefs of a client's culture. Cultural awareness involves also the examination of possible ethnocentrism in the practitioner's own values and beliefs. In addition, Campinah-Bacote advocates 'cultural desire', which is 'the motivation of the health care professional to "want" to engage in the process of cultural competence'. She argues that, although health care providers might be culturally aware, and possess knowledge and skill, without a full commitment to incorporate these into caring, these become meaningless.

Whether these kinds of ideas transfer very well to the microstructure of communicative events themselves however is problematic. Hart et al. (2003) argue that despite claims that students are taught to practise in antidiscriminatory or anti-oppressive ways, their work suggests that this may not yield practitioners who live out this model in their clinical work. Indeed, it may be a particularly unrealistic expectation in the case of preregistration students, who may still be preoccupied with acquiring basic clinical competencies and who may feel relatively powerless within the practice environment. Hart and colleagues advocate the development of what they call an 'inequalities imagination' which will allow practitioners in training to think their way into work with clients so as to take account of differences in background and lifestyle and which respects human rights and dignity. This helps make explicit the process of thinking about one's current practice and awareness of how they work with disadvantaged clients, and how they prepare others to do so.

The solution to building trust and effective communication between different ethnic, cultural and linguistic groups so that health care can be undertaken in an appropriate and sensitive manner is not easy. It requires ingenuity and an ability to think outside the box on the part of practitioners and indeed clients. In the UK there are many tales of how children of non-English speakers have to act as translators to mediate between their parents and health professionals.

The difficulty in bridging different worlds of experience, language and culture in health care and some solutions to help deal with this divide have been discussed by Greenhalgh et al. (2005) who describe an intervention to develop and refine a means of support and education for patients with diabetes in minority ethnic groups, delivered through bilingual health advocates, with particular focus on people of Bangladeshi extraction. Their previous research had shown that positive behaviour changes in Bangladeshi clients in the UK were almost always attributed by them to a story told in an informal setting by another Bangladeshi. Their study of diabetes care was intended to develop an intervention based on informal storytelling and evaluate its acceptability and subjective benefits to patients and staff. The community group where this was undertaken resisted formal models of group working where there is a facilitator and people take turns in telling their stories. However, there were many opportunities for sharing experience and reflecting on the lessons in these experiences for the question of 'what to do about diabetes?'. Alongside resistance to formal facilitation and a preagreed agenda, the stories are often fragmented and were sometimes enacted rather than told. From the facilitators' point of view however, the important point about these social events was the shared process of reacting to the story and discussing different interpretations and possible endings, which led to reflective learning and empowerment to take action. Stories emerged rather like the one below which we quote in its entirety.

The story of Mrs Uddin

This is an example of a client's story written up by a bilingual health advocate (from a themed session on 'diabetes in the family'):

> Mrs Uddin is a 35-year-old Bengali woman. She is 20 weeks pregnant and already has three children. Mrs Uddin recently came to this country and was diagnosed with diabetes. She had to face many difficulties. She was missing her family in Bangladesh. Her husband works outside London and visits twice a week. She therefore stays with her in-laws. Mrs Uddin was expecting her husband to take her to the GP. She was feeling very tired. When she eventually saw the midwife she found out she was diabetic. She had to start taking insulin for which she was dependent on others. Her grandmother and father had also been diabetic. Her father had not taken care of his health and he died at the age of 50.
>
> (Greenhalgh et al. 2005: 630)

Learning she was insulin dependent was frightening for Mrs Uddin and caused her to become depressed. She did not understand why she had to take insulin and thought it might cause her to die like her father. Due to language barriers that existed, Mrs Uddin found it difficult to get the necessary help when she needed it. She relied on her sister-in-law to inject her with insulin, but she often had to wait long lengths of time for her medication as her sister-in-law was busy. Mrs Uddin had been to the hospital a few times. The linkworker and health advocate had been regularly monitoring her progress and feeding back the information to the health professionals.

Why did you choose this story?

Because of the many difficulties Mrs Uddin had to face being diagnosed with diabetes away from home.

What questions or issues does this story raise?

Through the advocates Mrs Uddin realized that not taking her insulin properly would result in detrimental effects on her unborn baby.

What are the learning points?

Mrs Uddin became much more responsible for her own health and had more help from her extended family once they had gained knowledge about the condition and how to treat it. Mrs Uddin did not previously understand diabetes and found it difficult to treat herself. After being advised by the linkworker and health advocate, Mrs Uddin realized the seriousness of her condition and sorted out taking her medication regularly.

Tutor's feedback to the learning group about this story

This story illustrates a number of issues common in a family with diabetes. First, there is a positive family history and a 'horror story' of a relative with early death. Second, the family members with previous experience of caring for diabetes are not the ones who are around when a new case is diagnosed (in this case, because they are back in Bangladesh). Third, contrary to the popular stereotype, the support from this Asian extended family is inadequate – those who are competent to help also have their own lives to lead. Finally, there is a strong suggestion of both guilt and despair in the diabetic member: she is dependent on her relatives but also conscious of being a burden to them (reproduced from the *Sharing Stories* workbook, in Greenhalgh et al. 2005: 630).

As a result of having participated in the process with group members and advocates, Greenhalgh and colleagues noted that group participation achieved positive outcomes not solely through acquisition of knowledge, but by creating a social space in which participants could renegotiate the meaning of knowledge, and where action could be planned and discussed. While education is often assumed to involve transmitting knowledge from experts to learners, Greenhalgh and her colleagues discovered that both the advocates and the user groups spent a good deal of time repeatedly discussing knowledge, reframing and challenging it and thereby making it meaningful for the participants. As Freire (1974: 52) put it: 'Knowledge emerges only through invention and reinvention, through the restless, impatient, continuing, hopeful inquiry men [sic] pursue in the world, with the world, and with each other'. In addition, Denning (2000) notes the 'powerful link' between storytelling in group situations and subsequent action by participants.

Thus, these kinds of storytelling and sharing approaches have some important potentials to overcome the difficulties of intercultural or interethnic communication that have been noted by other authors. Also worth noting is the difference in approach here. Whereas many attempts made to characterize the situation faced by ethnic minorities and migrants, tell people about 'ethnic cultures' as if they were a series of facts to learn and try to give health care professionals more positive attitudes, Greenhalgh and colleagues's work suggests a way of working that enables people to learn about one another and solve problems in a dynamic way. This way of working is sensitive to changes in culture and differences between client groups without imposing a blanket definition of what it means to be a member of an 'ethnic minority'.

Bad news: delivering difficult information

Breaking bad news to clients or patients is a task which many health care professionals approach apprehensively. There is a considerable risk of upset to all concerned, as well as a likelihood of complaint or litigation. Until recently many doctors took the approach that the truth might be too much for the patient to bear, damaging to the therapeutic process, and therefore it was deemed preferable not to tell patients that they had, for example, cancer, and glossed over diagnoses of feared conditions such as multiple sclerosis with references to vague complaints such as 'neuritis'. Recently, as a result of a growing awareness of patients' rights to the medical information pertaining to their case, whether it be good or bad, practitioners have increasingly felt the obligation to deliver this news sensitively, skillfully and accurately (Gillotti and Applegate 2000).

As Douglas Maynard (2003:2) puts it: 'Bad news and good news are pervasive features of everyday life and experience. Waiting for, and then receiving, the news can send a recipient through cycles of dread, despair, depression, hope, elation, ecstasy, and other emotional states'.

Maynard struggles to define the 'common core' that he sees as central to news giving and receiving activities. Such news 'momentarily interrupts our involvement in the social world whose contours we otherwise unthinkingly accept as we carry on with daily activities' (p. 4).

On the face of it, in many news-giving encounters in health care there appears little for the analyst to see or do. As Maynard reports: 'I have recurrently witnessed physicians and other experts from internal medicine, oncology, developmental disability and HIV clinics present the tidings to patients or family members, who say nothing or, if they say something, it is very little and spoken in a resigned way' (p. 153–4).

As Cicourel (2005) adds, often patients and family members also do nothing, sitting rather rigidly in their chairs. This may be to do with the nature of this experience. Getting bad news may be bad for one's future life expectations, but it may also be a less than propitious clinical experience too. Thus, unlike other experiences such as joy or excitement there may be few immediate outward signs. It may also be that deliveries of bad news are themselves rather brief and offer few opportunities for extended interaction, which might be postponed to subsequent interactions. In one early study Cunningham and Sloper (1977) found that 64 per cent of parents of children with Down syndrome received a disclosure of the diagnosis which they felt was brief and inadequate. Based on the experience of two families, these early researchers portrayed a news-giving experience that appeared to them to be highly insensitive and disrespectful, which is bitterly remembered. Later, Sloper and Turner (1993) found that parental unhappiness at the way in which diagnoses were given remained high at 51 per cent, with 37 per cent of parents expressing severe dissatisfaction.

Thus, the delivery of bad news is an area where more sensitive handling and communicative skill might be desirable. It may be that there is no easy way to deliver bad news – because of the nature of the experience it is unlikely that anyone will be very pleased to receive it. Nevertheless the way in which it is delivered can add to the trauma. From the professionals' point of view, some recommend that the best way to learn how to do this is to observe senior colleagues breaking bad news (James 2001). In terms of the technique deployed, some have advocated that, given the impossibility of breaking bad news without causing distress, it should be given in a straightforward and direct manner (Essex 2001; Nolan 2001). Both these suggestions are open to doubt. Senior colleagues, despite their experience, would not necessarily have developed the skills which can fruitfully be copied – this may simply reproduce the very practices that clients complain about. Equally, even experienced clinicians express disquiet at having to do this sort of thing. For example, a survey reported by Ramirez et al. (1995) undertaken with non-surgical oncologists found that almost 50 per cent of respondents felt that they had insufficient training in communication skills, which was associated with higher stress scores, compared with those who reported that they had received sufficient training.

The experience of delivering bad news is one with which care providers are frequently faced, yet are often unsuccessful. Practitioners experience discomfort in such situations, and are left with a sense that they could somehow have done better (Bowers 1999). They are believed by many researchers to not deliver the bad news very effectively in most cases (Roth and Nelson 1997; Vetto 1999).

Perhaps it is worth noting that, as Gillotti et al. (2002) point out, the criteria for communicative competence in delivering bad news differ from the skills needed in the traditional medical consultation (McNeilis 2001). In the usual style of medical interviews, the success of information exchange sequences is likely to depend on skill and relational competence (Gilloti et al. 2002). This is believed to be especially true when practitioners are trying to verify information and follow up on topics that have been initiated by the patient. Some research suggests that the more competent practitioners communicate more information about diagnoses, prognoses and treatment options (McNeilis 2001). Consultation interviews may include a good deal of relationally oriented statements, humour and legitimizing affect than is typically found in bad news contexts (Gillotti et al. 2002).

Bad news on the other hand requires a somewhat different approach. Some ideas from the literature have been condensed by Fujimori et al. (2005) These include the desirability of having other health care professionals present when disclosing bad news, giving the patient the diagnosis only after it has been confirmed rather than while it is still speculative, informing the patient of the diagnosis honestly but not bluntly, sitting close to the patient to facilitate physical contact, and using lay language but without euphemisms.

In Fujimori et al.'s (2005) study of patients' preferences in being given bad news, participants preferred not to be given only the bad news. Instead they desired an opportunity to discuss the status of the disease, the possible treatment, and other related matters. In the case of cancer, participants made statements such as 'During the consultation I prefer to be told the stage of the cancer, its treatability, the cure rate for the cancer, and cancer-specific information' (p. 1046). Patients also described how they appreciated being given information that would give them hope. Many participants also expressed a preference for information about the impact of the disease and its treatments on their daily activities, especially their working lives. As Maynard (2003: 4) says, such news 'interrupts our involvement in the social world whose contours we otherwise unthinkingly accept as we carry on with daily activities' and participants are perhaps keen to repair this 'interruption'.

As a result of this investigation of patients' preferences, Fujimori et al. (2005: 1047) make some further recommendations, to the effect that practitioners should use supportive expressions which they believe will help relieve the patient's distress and offer reassurance, such as 'Don't worry. I'm on your side', 'Let's do our best together', and 'I promise to continue to see you'. Moreover, practitioners should allow patients to express their feelings and accept them.

The delivery of bad and good news is, according to Maynard (2003: 212) often asymmetric. One of the key differences is that 'it is as if bad new worlds just happen, while good new worlds are something we achieve'. Moreover professionals with bad news seek to 'eviscerate displays of their agency and responsibility' while 'professionals with good news work to display their agency and to claim responsibility' while trying to avoid 'possible attributions of self-praise' (p. 219).

In the delivery of news then, a complex management of identity and agency is undertaken by practitioners. Modestly claiming responsibility for favourable developments and avoiding blame for unfavourable ones is part of this complex dance of delivery. Thus, in Maynard's view, news delivery and receipt are not simply a matter of the 'social construction' of a particular problem or condition in any obvious sense. He reminds us that the participants are actively making and unmaking their world *in situ* in the interaction. This new world is not merely a verbal construction but involves the interactants' bodies, the social structures within which they are embedded and interactional events which yield not just words but manifestly 'real' social consequences. To the young woman recovering from the aftermath of an abusive and injurious sexual encounter, the diabetes sufferer in a language community she or he barely understands, or the person about to assume the identity of a 'cancer patient', the events concerned have an insistent 'reality' which is not easily captured by the term 'social construction'. In the light of this perhaps the best plan for the practitioner is to enter this reality and see what it looks like from the point of view of the client, so as to gauge how they would best like to proceed.

Conclusion: delicate matters

We have in this chapter provided a necessarily brief account of some of the contours of the discussion of difficult and delicate matters in health care contexts. Despite our attempts to provide detail and depth concerning studies, ideas and theories, we are aware that there is still precious little by way of sound advice for the newly qualified or experienced practitioner, and that once again the material available yields little more than we already would have known from experience of talking to friends and family. However, perhaps that is the key feature. While it is possible to create a summarized list of good practice points, we need to take on board Maynard's (2003) contention that the meanings of events are orchestrated through the participants building a new world through the nuances of interaction. In this light perhaps the best course of action to practitioners is to utilise reasonable guidance yet to be aware that little is fixed in this area. A warm, accepting attitude may be as useful as the mastery of protocols, even if we could agree upon a single model of best practice. The ability to work sensitively and empathically with clients may be easy to encourage but, in the face of other institutional constraints, be difficult to sustain in practice.

Equally, it is clear that there is far more at stake in many health care environments than simply the practitioner and the client. The situational constraints, other agencies involved, test results that do not come through, colleagues who are themselves overworked or on sick leave, arcane bureaucratic systems that are changed so frequently that no one knows how they are supposed to work, all have an impact on the situation faced by clients and practitioners. Indeed, the most commonsensical advice about good practice in communicating about sensitive issues is difficult to follow when faced with such frustrations. The delivery and receipt of bad news may be coloured by this knowledge of organized health and social care which participants bring to the situation. Knowing that help will be available in the future is very different from knowing otherwise. The growing confidence that some activists and clinicians have in antiretroviral drugs means that for some at least an HIV positive diagnosis is rather different now from what it might have meant a decade ago, for example.

The sensitivity of an issue, the 'badness' of the news or the delicacy which is deemed to be necessary depends a great deal on the social context. A clinical example from a colleague in practice illustrates this. She was visited one day by two elderly parents and their adult son. The family had recently migrated to the UK from northern Pakistan and the young man's behaviour had begun to give cause for concern. His eyes were downcast, he had a shuffling gait and did not respond to greetings or questions. Suspecting an underlying neurological problem our colleague referred him for further investigations by a neurologist. When the results came through and she met again with the family, she had some bad news to deliver. The son had developed Parkinson's disease at a tragically young age. Upon hearing this, the parents wept, but on subsequent enquiry it turned out that this was out of relief not sadness. They had feared that their son had become disabled as a result of copulating with the livestock in the old country, and according to local belief this would lead to the person concerned developing the characteristics of the animals in question. As a consequence, they felt that much shame attached to the young man and the family as a whole. Having a legitimate clinical diagnosis for the situation occasioned a great deal of relief. The sensitivities, then, may not always be quite what we expect.

References

Alexander, C., Edwards, R., Temple, B. et al. (2004) *Access to Services with Interpreters: User Views*. York: Joseph Rowntree Foundation.

Allan, K. and Burridge, K. (1991) *Euphemism and Dysphemism: Language Used as Shield and Weapon*. New York: Oxford University Press.

Bakhtin, M.M. (1986) *Speech Genres and Other Late Essays*, in C. Emerson and M. Holquist (eds and translators) Austin, TX: University of Texas Press.

Bergstrom, L., Roberts, J., Skillman, L. and Seidel, J. (1992) 'You'll feel me touching you, sweetie': vaginal examinations during the second stage of labour, *Birth*, 19(1): 10–18.

Bhatia, V.K. (1993) *Analyzing Genre: Language Use in Professional Settings*. London: Longman.

Bowers, L.J. (1999) Back to basics ... 'I've got some bad news . . .', *Topics in Clinical Chiropractics*, 6(1–8): 69–71.

British Medical Association (2005) *Sexual Health June 2005*. Available at http://www.bma.org.uk/ap.nsf/Content/sexualhealthjune05 (accessed 13 March 2006).

Brown, P. and Levinson, S.C. (1987) *Politeness*. New York: Cambridge University Press.

Campinah-Bacote, J. (1999) A model and instrument for addressing cultural competence in health care, *Journal of Nursing Education*, 38: 202–7.

Cicourel, A. (2005) Review of Maynard, D. (2003) Bad news, good news, *Language in Society*, 34: 282–91.

Cooper, C.R. and Denner, J. (1998) Theories linking culture and psychopathology: universal and community-specific processes, *Annual Review of Psychology*, 49: 559–84.

Cooper, L.A. and Roter, D.L. (2003) Patient–provider communication: the effect of race and ethnicity on process and outcomes of health care, in B.D. Smedley, A.Y. Stith and A.R. Nelson (eds) *Unequal Treatment: Confronting Racial and Ethnic Disparities in Health Care*. Washington, DC: National Academy Press.

Cunningham, C.C. and Sloper, P. (1977) Parents of Down's syndrome babies: their early needs, *Child Care, Health and Development*, 3: 325–47.

Denning, S. (2000) *The Springboard: How Storytelling Ignites Action in Knowledge-era Organizations*. New York: Butterworth-Heinemann.

Dustmann, C., Fabbri, F., Preston, I. and Wadsworth, J. (2003) *The Labour Market Performance of Immigrants in the UK Labour Market*. Home Office Report 05/03. London: Home Office.

Emerson, J. (1971) Behaviour in private places: sustaining definitions of reality in gynaecological examinations, in H. Dreitzel (ed.) *Recent Sociology No. 2*. London: Macmillan.

Essex, C. (2001) Delivering bad news: Receiving bad news will always be unpleasant, *British Medical Journal*, 322: 864–5.

Ewick, P. and Silbey, S.S. (1995) Subversive stories and hegemonic tales: toward a sociology of narrative, *Law and Society*, 29(2): 197–226.

Fowler, A. (1989) Genre, in E. Barnouw (ed.) *International Encyclopedia of Communications*, Vol. 2. New York: Oxford University Press.

Friere, P. (1974) *Education for Critical Consciousness*. New York: Continuum.

Fujimori, M., Akechi, T., Akizuki, N. et al. (2005) Good communication with patients receiving bad news about cancer in Japan, *Psycho-Oncology*, 14: 1043–51.

Gillotti, C.M. and Applegate, J.L. (2000) Explaining illness as bad news: individual differences in explaining illness-related information, in B. Whaley (ed.) *Explaining Illness*. Mahwah, NJ: Lawrence Erlbaum Associates.

Gillotti, C.M., Thompson, T. and McNeilis, K. (2002) Communicative competence in the delivery of bad news, *Social Science and Medicine*, 54: 1011–23.

Glazener, C.M.A. (1997) Sexual function after childbirth: women's experiences, persistent morbidity and lack of professional recognition, *British Journal of Obstetrics and Gynaecology*, 104: 330–5.

Greenhalgh, T., Collard, A. and Begum, N. (2005) Sharing stories: complex intervention for who do not speak English: diabetes education in minority ethnic groups, *British Medical Journal*, 330: 628–34.

Grossen, M. and Apotheloz, D. (1998) Intelligence as a sensitive topic in clinical interviews prompted by learning difficulties, *Pragmatics*, 8(2): 239–54.

Hart, A., Hall, V. and Henwood, F. (2003) Helping health and social care professionals to develop an 'inequalities imagination': a model for use in education and practice, *Journal of Advanced Nursing*, 41(5): 480–9.

James, A. (2001) Hearing the worst, *Guardian*, 25 April.

Johnson, R. and Taylor, W. (2000) *Skills for Midwifery Practice*. Edinburgh: Churchill Livingstone.

Johnson, R.I., Saha, S., Arbelaez, J.J., Beach, M.C. and Cooper, L.A. (2004) Racial and ethnic differences in patient perceptions of bias and cultural competence in health care, *Journal of General Internal Medicine*, 19: 101–10.

Karlsen, S. and Nazroo, J.Y. (2002) Agency and structure: the impact of ethnic identity and racism on the health of ethnic minority people, *Sociology of Health and Illness*, 24(1): 1–20.

Krieger, N. and Sidney, S. (1996) Racial discrimination and blood pressure: the CARDIA Study of Young Black Adults, *American Journal of Public Health*, 86(10): 1370–8.

Laqueur, T.W. (2003) *Solitary Sex: A Cultural History of Masturbation*. New York: Zone Books.

LaVeist, T. (1996) Why we should continue to study race . . . but do a better job: an essay on race, racism and health, *Ethnicity and Disease*, 6: 21–9.

Lavender, T. and Walkinshaw, S.A. (1998) Can midwives reduce postpartum psychological morbidity? A randomized trial, *Birth*, 25: 215–19.

Lawler, J. (1991) *Behind the Screens: Nursing, Somology, and the Problem of the Body*. Edinburgh: Churchill Livingstone.

McNeilis, K.L. (2001) Analyzing communication competence in medical consultation, *Health Communication*, 13: 5–18.

Maynard, D. (2003) *Bad News, Good News: Conversational Order in Everyday Talk and Clinical Settings*. Chicago: University of Chicago Press.

Nolan, P.C. (2001) Not all surgeons can counsel, and fewer psychotherapists can operate (letter), *British Medical Journal*, 322: 865.

Parekh, B. (2000) *The Future of Multi-ethnic Britain: The Report of the Commission on the Future of Multi-ethnic Britain* (the Parekh Report). London: Profile Books.

Pitts, M. (1996) *The Psychology of Preventive Health*. London: Routledge.

Preston, G. (2005) *At Greatest Risk: The Children Most Likely to Be Poor*. London: Child Poverty Action Group.

Ramirez, A.J., Graham, J., Richards, M. et al. (1995) Burnout and psychiatric disorder among cancer clinicians, *British Journal of Cancer*, 71(6): 1263–9.

Roth, N.L. and Nelson, M.S. (1997) HIV diagnosis rituals and identity narratives, *AIDS Care*, 9: 161–79.

Schiffrin, D. (1994) *Approaches to Discourse*. Cambridge, MA: Blackwell.

Schulman, K.A., Berlin, J.A. and Harless, W. (1999) The effect of race and sex on physicians' recommendations for cardiac catheterization. *New England Journal of Medicine*, 340: 618–26.

Serrant-Green, L. (2005) Breaking traditions: sexual health and ethnicity in nursing research: a literature review, *Journal of Advanced Nursing*, 51(5): 511–19.

Shaw, C., Williams, K.S. and Assassa, R.P. (2000) Patients' views of a new nurse-led continence service, *Journal of Clinical Nursing*, 9: 574–84.

Shildrick, M. (1997) *Leaky Bodies and Boundaries: Feminism, Postmodernism and (Bio)ethics*. London: Routledge.

Sloper, P. and Turner, S. (1993) Determinants of parental satisfaction with disclosure of disability, *Developmental Medicine and Child Neurology*, 35: 816–25.

Smedley, B.D., Stith, A.Y. and Nelson, A.R. (eds) (2003) *Unequal Treatment: Confronting Racial and Ethnic Disparities in Health Care*. Washington, DC: National Academy Press.

Stewart, M. (2005) 'I'm just going to wash you down': sanitizing the vaginal examination, *Journal of Advanced Nursing*, 51(6): 587–94.

Swales, J.M. (1990) *Genre Analysis*. Cambridge: Cambridge University Press.

Taylor, J.S. (2003) Confronting 'culture' in medicine's 'culture of no culture', *Academic Medicine*, 78: 555–9.

Thakar, R. and Sultan, A.H. (2003) Management of obstetric anal sphincter injury, *Obstetrician Gynaecologist*, 5(2): 72–8.

Trinch, S.L. (2001) Managing euphemism and transcending taboos: negotiating the meaning of sexual assault in Latinas' narratives of domestic violence, *Text*, 21(4): 567–610.

Twigg, J. (2000) *Bathing: The Body and Community Care*. London: Routledge.

US Department of Health and Human Services (USDHHS) (1999) *Mental Health: A Report of the Surgeon General*. Rockville, MD: US Department of Health and Human Services, Public Health Service, Office of the Surgeon General.

van Ryn, M. and Burke, J. (2000) The effect of patient race and socio-economic status on physicians' perceptions of patients, *Social Science and Medicine*, 50: 813–28.

van Ryn, M. and Fu, S.S. (2003) Paved with good intentions: do public health and human service providers contribute to racial/ethnic disparities in health? *American Journal of Public Health*, 93: 248–50.

Vetto, J.T. (1999) Teaching medical students to give bad news: does formal instruction help? *Journal of Cancer Education*, 14: 13–17.

Wear, D. (2003) Insurgent multiculturalism: rethinking how and why we teach culture in medical education, *Academic Medicine*, 78: 549–54.

Williams, A., Lavender, T., Richmond, D. and Tincello, D.G. (2005) Women's experiences after a third-degree obstetric anal sphincter tear: a qualitative study, *Birth*, 32(2): 129–36.

Zhou, M. and Bankston, C.L. (1998) *Growing up American: How Vietnamese Children Adapt to Life in the United States*. Thousand Oaks, CA: Sage.

9 Health education and communication: changing, informing, compliance and concordance

Health communication and cultural context

Many threats to human health are difficult to ameliorate. Problems such as heart disease, cancer and HIV infection are difficult to cure in any simple sense, so hopes have been pinned on the potential of health education, for example, through campaigns to reduce smoking, increase the uptake of exercise and safer sex practices or to facilitate early diagnoses through screening and testing. Yet at the same time there are concerns that many lavishly funded campaigns have had limited effectiveness or that as much as half of the medication paid for from the steadily increasing UK drugs bill is not taken as directed, thus reducing its likely therapeutic effect. This chapter examines scholarship in health language and communication that offers new insights into how health education might work better and how changes in communication strategies may bridge the gap between professional and lay perspectives or even enhance compliance within a spirit of concordance.

In some parts of the world, for example Australasia, notions of health promotion have been tied in with grander social concerns such as social justice, anti-harassment policies and an inclusive approach to decision making in the institutions where health was promoted. Making sense of effective health promotion campaigns then is about far more than merely examining attitude changes. In other parts of the world, such as the USA, the discourse of health promotion is intimately connected with discourses about the self, the individual's personality and their sense of self-efficacy. Indeed, the language of health promotion involves a range of discourses about wider institutional and political contexts.

Given such diversity we shall not be able to cover all the aspects of health promotion and communication in this chapter. Instead we will reduce our focus to tease out how we can add to our understanding of the meaning of health-related communications. We will attempt to indicate some of the complexities of undertaking evaluating health promotion via studies into accounts of smoking and sexual health, much of which has been focused on children and young people. Finally, we will then go on more generally to examine compliance and concordance, an issue with major implications across the life cycle.

Smoking: cultures, communities and the difficulties of cutting down

The prevalence of smoking, especially among young people remains higher than many health educators would like it to be (Johnston et al. 2003; Substance Abuse and Mental Health Services Administration [SAMHSA] 2003). The UK is fairly typical of industrialized and post industrial nations in that 28 per cent of males and 24 per cent of females are believed to be regular smokers. Among young adults the prevalence is much higher, with over a fifth being regular smokers by the age of 15 and rates of smoking among 20–24-year-olds being 36 per cent. Among younger people, women are slightly more likely to smoke than men (Office for National Statistics 2003, 2004; Cancer Research UK 2005).

Despite the well documented hazards attached to smoking (Doll and Hill 1950; US Department of Health and Human Services [USDHHS] 2001; Johnson and Richter 2002) and the massive investments in health education campaigns by many governments, health care and charitable bodies, smoking remains stubbornly popular, and is usually commenced in adolescence. Beyond the major physical health consequences of this early start, there are a wide range of associated psychosocial problems in younger people, such as poor academic performance, drug and alcohol use, and delinquency (Escobedo et al. 1997; Ellickson et al. 2001; Tucker et al. 2006). Moreover, girls who smoke are disproportionately likely to experience early parenthood, by a factor of 5 to 1 (Ellickson et al. 2001). As has been noted, these impacts can result in social exclusion and difficult transitions to adult roles and responsibilities (Chassin et al. 2000; Orlando et al. 2004). In this context, devising health promotion materials for smokers will be especially challenging as these factors combine into an 'over-determined nexus' (Gabriel and Todorova 2003) which may be especially difficult to unpick as the different elements may sustain each other.

It is not our purpose here to review all the attempts to encourage young people not to smoke or assist people in giving up. There is a massive literature on this subject already. Rather, what we shall do is to identify some of the work which can be done using a fine-grained attention to language and social life so as to help us understand why the messages from the adult world, policymakers and health educators may be difficult for young people to take seriously. Perhaps, as we shall see, the cultures in which youngsters are embedded and the communicative practice they participate in might be seen to encourage smoking, with its desirability supervening over and above the messages about its negative effects. Unless we grasp these issues, it will be difficult to achieve the substantial reduction in smoking that is advocated by health educators and policymakers.

To explore the meaning of smoking, a study by Lucas and Lloyd (1999) compared three groups of girls who were about 13–14 years old: those who had never smoked; those who were regular smokers; and those who were experimental smokers. Girls who belonged to 'never smoked' groups had an identity which stressed that they were quiet, sensible and tended to stay in as opposed to going out. In describing themselves and others like them, they might say, for example:

I: Can you tell me why she's not the type to smoke?

R: I think she's too sensible

I: Too sensible. Does that mean people who smoke are stupid then?

R: Yeah (laugh)

I: OK, so F's sensible. What else about her?

R: I think cos she's quite quiet as well. I think cos she's a bit like me would rather just stay home watch the telly or laughs do something like that.

(p. 650)

Smokers were perceived to demand conformity in smoking behaviour and within groups of smokers there was often a description of how they initially started out as anti-smoking but changed their orientation:

> before I went round with you lot [friendship smoking group] I never smoked and everyone's going 'You're going to smoke in a year, I bet you next year you're going to be smoking' ... And then after that I thought 'I'm going to smoke' and like something happened, I can't remember what ... '
>
> (p. 654)

'Smokers are seen by their peers as fun loving and non-conformist and cigarettes as a passport to an exciting and popular lifestyle' (Lucas and Lloyd 1999: 654). The authors go on to say that it may prove difficult to create an alternative that has the same appeal as the social representations of the smoker identity.

This kind of identification and image of smoking was also apparent in a study in New Zealand by Plumridge et al. (2002). Participants said for example: 'On a sort of fashionable, cool basis, out of 10, you've got people who um, well, then you've got people like in our class who are like a one, or one and a half ... And then there are the smokers and they, um and you know are like ten (p. 170).

However, the relationship between smoking and social popularity and success was by no means inevitable. Whereas the more 'cool' or popular adolescents tended to smoke, some who did so still fell short. Indeed, smoking could be seen as a kind of desperate strategy adopted by some children to get themselves out of a devalued category and ascend the social hierarchy:

IntV: So he's a nerd but he smokes and, and why do you think he smokes?

Gary: 'Cos he doesn't want to look like a nerd.

Phil: Yeah.

IntV: But he can't escape being a nerd.

Phil: And he buys friendship. Like he goes out there and he gives people smokes.

(Plumridge et al. 2002: 171)

The material from Lucas and Lloyd (1999) and Plumridge et al. (2002) alerts us to the fact that there are a variety of lifestyle and social factors involved which health education campaigns must successfully address in order to persuade young people that smoking is not a good idea. There is a social idiom, or, in Bourdieu's sense, (1984 1990), 'habitus', of which smoking is often seen as an essential part. Some people and some social groups are much more attuned to the proximal cues of their immediate social matrix than they are to the health education messages which are seen to be dull but worthy and associated with an adult world which they are finding increasingly distant and irrelevant to their lives. This then is the kind of territory that can be explored through attending to the communicative activities which are unfolding within the groups most likely to take up smoking and between these people and interviewers. Rather than conceptualize the issue in terms of 'peer pressure', it might be productive to formulate the issue instead in terms of the linguistic and subcultural factors involved in forming and performing identities.

The appeal of smoking to young adults also relates to other drugs of choice among this generation, not least cannabis (Clark et al. 2002; Fraser 2002). Among 15-year-olds surveyed in Scotland 34 per cent of boys and 30 per cent of girls reported that they had used cannabis, with around a fifth reporting use in the last month (Boreham and Shaw 2001). Concerns have been raised about how the popularity and increased access to the drug might have health and social consequences, especially for respiratory health (British Lung Foundation 2002; Drummond 2002; Henry et al. 2003), and the inter-relationship between smoking tobacco and the use of cannabis (Amos et al. 2004). In the latter study, participants tended to describe the use of cannabis pre-dating and encouraging the use of tobacco:

> I used to smoke hash then when I couldn't get it or didn't have it I smoked fags. (focus group males C2DE)

> When I went up to college I hadn't smoked at all, but then I was in the social scene of like smoking hash and things like that, I got into that and then that made me get addicted to tobacco. (interviews F99 unemployed)
>
> (Amos et al. 2004: 79)

How the possession of cigarettes was implicated – indeed necessary – for the cannabis smoker was described in the focus group part of Amos and colleagues's study:

> Like you really just use the fag to roll a joint and if you've no' got any hash, you just smoke your fags. (focus group males ABC1)

> P: You smoke both really because somebody will go 'Aye, give me a fag for a joint' and then you'll give them a fag and then
> Int: You swap a fag for a joint?
> P: Aye, they still need to roll it and then you tend to have like a fag while waiting on them rolling it. (focus group males C2DE)
>
> (p. 79)

This suggests that the use of tobacco is built into the social situation of drug taking. Indeed, a recent US community study found that adult smokers who used cannabis were much less likely to have quit smoking 13 years later than non-users (Ford et al. 2002). Thus, there is some evidence that those using cannabis regularly have more incentive to carry on smoking.

Researchers have investigated the incidence or prevalence of smoking or drug taking in a large variety of qualitative and quantitative studies. Indeed, such is the topic exposure that for many young people, as Parker et al. (2002) put it, in their grandly titled 'normalization thesis', recreational drug use is relatively 'normal' and is not considered to be remarkable or reprehensible by increasing sections of the population. Yet from the point of view of social science itself, there is a good deal more that could yet be achieved. The few examples presented earlier come from a much larger body of social and educational literature documenting the practices and attitudes of the teenage smoker or drug taker, supplemented locally in many health authority prevalence studies.

In the light of this, we would argue that what is needed are more attempts to ground this well-developed field of enquiry in a more far reaching understanding of the process of being an adolescent in contemporary societies, given the social stresses and uncertainties that are often believed to be influential on youngsters. It is sometimes suggested that it is difficult being a young adult in a world which does not appear to enjoy a 'moral consensus' or where political ambivalence is endemic (Mouffe 2005) or where, as a number of thinkers like Beck (1992) contend, people may have high psychological, educational and material expectations, but face the experience of fragmented families and communities and minimum-wage employment opportunities.

Thus rather than simply cataloguing prevalence and attitudes, we would argue for the need to understand the smoking and drug-taking activities of participants as part of a more comprehensive set of lifestyles, embedded in a complex of social, moral and ideological frameworks or 'habitus'. This includes practices and schemes of perception, preference and taste acquired over time and which are themselves informed by internalizations of material life chances. This relates also to the question of what young people comprehend of the society we now live in as well as the social cliques at school, and could lead to the creation of some interesting, theoretically informed evidence-based accounts of local cultures and communication patterns which would offer some new ideas for effective health-promotion campaigns.

There are already some hints that this is happening. Following on from the work of Bourdieu, Poland et al. (2006) argue that it is better to address the social contexts of smoking in adolescence – the deeper structuring of the alignment of material life chances, social position and styles of living which characterize social groups, communities of taste, shared dispositions, ways of life, and images of social identity. In this view it is considerably more than a set of mediating variables explaining individual choice. This represents a new way of understanding behaviour as a kind of routinized and socialized pattern of consumption which is meaningful and common to particular groups.

Poland et al. (2006) stress the need for researchers to address the issue of power relations and the central importance of place and time in smoking behaviour, for example behind the bicycle shed, the pub or amidst the post-coital afterglow. So far there is little in the way of studies providing a systematic and comprehensive basis for understanding the social embeddedness of collective social practices. Bridging this gap involves attending to the profoundly local contexts of discourse about smoking and linking them to the social world so as to guide researchers and health educators in conceptualizing the relationship between smoking and social context.

Poland et al. (2006) also introduce a plea for greater reflexivity in the work of tobacco use control, encouraging researchers to break with the assumptions of pre-dictability, certainty and potential controllability that characterize a modernist emphasis on evidence-based best practice and adopt a self-critical, postmodern atti-tude so as to question rigorously taken-for-granted assumptions regarding the political nature of health education work, its effects and how these effects may have different impacts on different social groups (Ruch 2002; Maton 2003).

Moreover, as Poland et al. (2006) remind us, there is an urgent need to understand how conventional smoking-reduction initiatives may unintentionally compound other forms of social exclusion in marginalized groups of people. Indeed, current practice may be generating resistance to anti-smoking publicity, and may partly be responsible for how some groups become 'hard to reach'. There may be an increasing mismatch in fundamental assumptions, 'life-worlds', lived experiences or habitus between middle-class professionals and their socially excluded 'clientele'. It is the study of discourse and social context which may help us bridge that gap and grasp the role smoking or drug taking play in the life-worlds of those who indulge in these pastimes. This way we can begin to understand the value of these activities for those involved, and health edu-cators can begin to devise approaches that lead to people adopting more effective health practices, rather than deepening the divisions which currently separate the worlds of youngsters from those of health promoters and educators.

The study of communication and meaning surrounding sex is another good example of how the worlds of educators and health promoters and the social and moral landscapes of the young people they are trying to communicate with can often be deeply divided.

Sex: navigating through hazardous territory

A focus on sex by health communicators, educators and policymakers has often been prompted by public health and epidemiological concerns in Europe, Australasia and North America (Evans and Tripp 2006). According to the UK's Health Protection Agency (2003), the incidence of sexually transmitted infections (STIs) among young people is increasing in England, Wales and Northern Ireland, and teenage pregnancy rates in England and Wales have been considered the highest in western Europe (Social Exclusion Unit 1992; Wilson and Huntington 2005). Despite a belief in earlier times that the teenage years are most appropriate for childbearing (Walker et al. 1976) and that becoming a parent over the age of 30 was problematic, contemporary policy-makers and educators believe that effective interventions need to be developed to reduce teenage pregnancy; ironically these are most fervently expressed in countries with an already declining birthrate. In line with what we have discussed concerning smoking and tobacco control, evidence suggests that interventions enjoy greater effectiveness when tailored to the different sexual attitudes and behaviour between the sexes and diverse ethnic groups (Connell et al. 2004). One aspect of this attempt to reach particular intended audiences involves trying to make the language and issues addressed meet the needs, levels of understanding and concerns of the target group (Dicenso et al. 2002; OFSTED 2002).

In addition to devising and testing messages and modes of delivery, then, some researchers have suggested that these can be shaped by the expertise of the target groups themselves. For example, Goold et al.'s (2006) participants suggested improving awareness of local genitourinary medicine services by the use of colourful advertisements; a range of media including computer games; placing information about services and how to access them in schools, colleges, youth clubs, on buses and at sports grounds; and by providing a 'virtual sexual health clinic' on the Internet.

In encouraging people to take care of their sexual health, Goold et al. (2006) suggest that it is more effective to foreground so called 'gain frames' where the benefits, for example, of using condoms or engaging in screening and detection practices, are given greater emphasis than the cost of not doing so ('loss frames'). For example, a 'gain-framed' message might appear as follows: 'By going to your local clinic you will benefit from advice from qualified staff, where you can collect free contraception (e.g. condoms) and advice leaflets'; whereas, a 'loss-framed' message would be: 'By not going to your local clinic you will miss out on the benefit from advice from qualified staff, and miss out on collecting free contraception (e.g. condoms) and advice leaflets' (p. 23).

Despite this confidence in designing messages to address young people's sexual health, pregnancy and exposure to risk, it should be noted that what is missing is an overall framework for making sense of the status of risk in young people's lives. Many authors have tried to make sense of young people's risk taking and the complex interplay of individual learning, decision making, identity and situated contexts of family, peers and community (e.g. Cohen and Ainley 2000; Lawy 2002). Young people are sometimes curiously protected from exposure to risk, yet also increasingly expected to manage their own reflexive life projects. Their learning and choice making are locally and structurally situated. According to Lawy: 'risk, identity and learning are mutually constitutive ... the challenge facing ... young people [is] to seam together risk, identity and learning within a coherent narrative, and to do so in the face of competing interests and structural limits in the knowledge that the balance between them might, at any moment, be changed' (2002: 407).

Once we begin to think about how sexuality is conceptualized, practised, negotiated and expressed we are reminded of the inadequacy of our notions of individual agency, desire or risk minimization when discussing sexual encounters. Alternatively, we might think of young people as being made up of distinct sexual personas, each attuned to the multiple social contexts they experience. Their actions in each context flow from a context-dependent disposition. Once again, Bourdieu's notion of 'habitus' is useful here, as a mechanism that 'ensures the active presence of past experiences, which, deposited in each organism in the form of schemes of perception, thought and action, tend to guarantee the "correctness" of practices and their constancy over time, more reliably than all formal rules and explicit norms' (1990: 41).

An example of this kind of habitus in a group of young people can be discerned in Hyde et al.'s (2005) study of people in their final years of school in Ireland and their feelings about sex education. While this group identified some common issues in their need for information, such as knowledge of STIs, the young men – in line with broader constructions of manhood – wanted more information on what they called the 'practical' issues around the mechanics of sex:

Int: Did you get sex education in school?
P4: Just … general knowledge (general laughter)
P3: There was no practical side to it! (general laughter)
(Male, Rural, Leaving Certificate, School 1 (Co-ed)/ Focus Group 1)

(p. 336)

Among the practical issues raised was their desire for information on using condoms correctly, and the suspicion that there was somehow more information dispensed to children in England. From the point of view of the young men in the study, their demands from sex education were largely centred on enhancing sexual performance. As Hyde et al. (2005) point out, this reinforces a dominant masculine identity that was already pervasive in young men's cultural milieu. This group wanted a particular kind of masculine identity to be enhanced and supported in sex education classes. Their desire to know more about putting condoms on is commendable from the point of view of health educators, but even so, in this case it seems to be bound up with the issue of perfecting performance in penetrative sex (Potts 2002).

To explore and exploit the opportunities offered by this kind of peer culture, health educators have frequently turned to 'peer tutoring' as an approach which can be used to deliver health promotion in the context of schools, colleges and youth work (Prince 1995; White and Pitts 1997; Svenson 1998; Frederick and Barlow 2006). The idea of peer education does not necessarily draw upon sociological theory, linguistics or pragmatics but instead is usually grounded in social psychological theories and ideas including Social Learning Theory, Diffusion of Innovation and Social Inoculation Theory (McGuire 1969; Bandura 1977; Rogers 1983).

Given that social influence is considered to be a key motivator of change, interpersonal communication is significant in securing attitude and behaviour change. Thus, over the last couple of decades, the issue of peer approaches to sex education has excited some interest. There is a widespread belief that traditional sex education has failed, as well as concern about the transmission of HIV, and also infections such as chlamydia and hepatitis. During this time it was discovered also that parents do not talk openly about this to their children and teachers are often embarrassed by the subject. On the other hand, from the early years of the twentieth century, the finding that young people learn about sex from their friends has been noted consistently by writers in this area (Exner 1915; Ramsay 1943; Schofield 1973). In an attempt to capitalize on this, there has been a rapid growth in 'peer education' schemes in Britain. From this perspective, young people are thus seen as an active resource rather than passive recipients of material from adults.

Conversations about sex and sexuality can cover a variety of content, from relationships and feelings through to descriptions of the activity itself, though as Walker (1997) notes, this is rare. Some people never have this kind of conversation with anyone. Such conversations could be informative or misleading, supportive or undermining. They may be entered into for a variety of reasons, including reputation maintenance, attempts to gain status, friendly support, the establishment of individuality (Heath 1982), amusement and gossip, as well as information gathering.

However, as Walker (1997) argues, there may be few opportunities for effective information transfer between peers. Certainly, there is much reported talk about sex but the conversations may have little content when it comes to useful information. As one informant said, 'We don't completely trust what they're saying 'cos no-one actually knows anything'. In particular Walker (1997) found that young men who had previously been boastful became silent when they had found regular partners. Maybe this was out of gallant loyalty to their partners or maybe because actual rather than mythical details of the sexual 'performance' could be compared. Moreover, it was difficult to find the right place and time for serious conversation: 'You can't just go up to someone and say, "I hear you've got this rash"', as one informant said (p. 50). Equally there was a fear of causing offence: 'If someone's got this new boyfriend or girlfriend and they're completely in love with them and you start saying, "Well, make sure you use a condom because they might be HIV positive," they feel really insulted' (p. 51). Moreover there was a suspicion that people outside their usual social circle wouldn't want to be seen talking to a peer educator as it would be assumed they had a problem.

The prospects for peer education, says Walker, are rather poor, because although most young people say they have learned most about sex from their friends, they find it very difficult to recall any facts they have learned in this way. It seems as if friends are used more as sounding boards for ideas or snippets of information. These are then assimilated into the picture or rejected depending on their 'fit' with an individual's picture of the world and their place in it (von Glasersfeld 1991).

The necessity of doing something about teenage sexuality and sexual knowledge has been pressing on the minds of policymakers and educators especially in the light of underage sex. According to the UK-based Brook Advisory Service (2002), the age at which young people report their first experience of sex is 14 years for women and 13 years for men. However, once attitudes and feelings are explored, women are more likely to report regretting it afterwards, saying they felt pressured into having intercourse and being more worried about pregnancy (De Gaston et al. 1996). The earliest experiences of sex are likely to fall short of full intercourse. A study in schools across one health authority in England found that 11 per cent of 13-year-olds surveyed had experienced full sexual intercourse (Burrack 1999).

Despite the concern this raises, combating sexual health-related problems might prove difficult. Studies show that professionals are not comfortable dealing with adolescent sexuality (Blum et al. 1996). Or, they may be disapproving. A study of providers of sexual health care to young people (Pitts et al. 1996: 1) discovered that 'all providers tended to hold negative views of young people and their sexual activity'. This may represent a missed opportunity, for, as Porter (2002) argues, these health care professionals could 'begin to understand and facilitate early adolescent females' healthy sexual development'.

There seems in many cases to be reluctance on the part of young people to talk about conscious experience during sex itself. Wight et al. (2000) found that 40 per cent of 13–14-year-olds who said they had had intercourse claimed to have been 'drunk or stoned' at the time. Poulin and Graham (2001) discovered that those who had unplanned sexual intercourse while under the influence of alcohol were disproportionately likely also to report multiple sexual partners and inconsistent condom use. As we are dealing with self-report surveys for the most part, we do not know whether blood alcohol levels were indeed high. What is interesting is that youngsters so regularly describe themselves as having been drunk. This might be coincidental, but it chimes in with other aspects of young people's sex talk that other scholars are beginning to disclose.

Mason (2005) undertook a study of advice workers who counsel youngsters about sexual health matters, and found a high level of concern that young people lack knowledge or awareness about sexual health and even what had happened to them:

> Now this is the most common one. They'll come in and go 'I don't know if I've actually had sex or not, but when I woke up my knickers were off or something and I feel a bit sore'. And that's the most typical one we get, where they don't know, they've trusted somebody and that's it, they don't know what they've done (Interview 7).
>
> (p. 201)

Or as others put it:

> They haven't a clue! You mention infection and they go 'oh'? Cause all they're worrying about is pregnancy. (Interview 1)
>
> Infections don't play a part in their brain at all! (Interview 7)
>
> You talk to them about infections and stuff and it's as though you are talking a foreign language to them. (Interview 8)
>
> (p. 202)

This apparent lack of information was a source of some puzzlement to the workers:

> You would think that they know everything about sex from what they read in magazines. It still surprises me how naïve [they are], in spite of all this. (Interview 2)
>
> (p. 203)

If youngsters are indeed not aware of sexuality and sexually transmitted infections and likely to be drunk at the time anyway, this has major implications for issues of sexual health and teen motherhood, especially as approaches to policy development are striving to be evidence-based (Mason 2005). In relation to this, many authors and researchers have taken very literally the idea that youngsters are naïve and not knowledgeable and have responded by ever more extensive and inventive forms of education. However, if we see the issue a little differently and think in terms of the relationship between language, knowledge and broader patterns of habitus and culture, a different explanation emerges, which is much more challenging for health educators.

In its cultural context, knowledge about sex, pregnancy and STIs, and even knowing about whether one has had sex oneself, is not an innocent kind of knowledge. If one knows too much about this kind of thing or talks too openly about having had sex, this can be problematic in many peer cultures, where sexualized insults can cut very deep indeed. The work of Lees (1993), Kitzinger (1995) and Stewart (1999) is instructive in that it shows how their informants were managing their identities within peer groups. For girls – who have been studied the most – there is often an intricate, complex and not always successful process of avoiding being thought of as a 'slag' (Cowie and Lees 1987; Lees 1993; Kitzinger 1995). In other parts of the world local idioms have their own sexual insults for young women, but here the term 'slag' or 'slut' was often used. The meaning of these terms has multiple layers. Most obviously they mean someone who has sex either too freely or without a suitable interval elapsing between partners, but on further exploration it is clear that the name-callers do not have firsthand knowledge of any actual sexual activity. The terms might mean someone who wears clothes too small for her, or is believed to be somehow unclean, or who lives in the wrong neighbourhood or is trying too hard to impress boys. In any case, there are considerable efforts expended by the young women in these studies to avoid being thought of as 'slags' or 'sluts'. Knowing too much about sex or STI prevention, talking about it, or describing oneself as having deliberately entered into sexual activity could put one at risk of being called a 'slag'.

According to Stewart (1999), young women may be caught up in a 'system of constraints and privations' (see also Foucault 1977: 11). Holland et al. (1996) suggest that young women's 'reputations' are constructed by their participants on an ongoing basis, and reflect a good many everyday values about what it means to be heterosexual and feminine. A young woman's reputation is very much a social construct; it does not necessarily reflect her actual sexual activity but is to do with how she acts, what she wears, how she diets and – crucially – what other people think of her.

The business of managing one's reputation, says Stewart (1999), is one aspect of securing their obedience to patriarchy (see Bartky 1990). This enlists young women in actively policing their own and others' behaviour. The young women in Stewart's study tended to point to young men in their peer groups as the principal originators of the judgment of some girls as 'sluts' or 'slags' but it could just as easily be applied by young women to one another.

We might speculate that this managing of reputation could be responsible for the difficulties in peer education schemes identified by Walker (1997) and the lack of awareness or knowledge described by Mason's (2005) informants. Looking at the context in which language or knowledge is used, then, and the forms of life or 'habitus' within which they are embedded can show us just what an uphill struggle health educators still have ahead of them. The challenge is to inform youngsters in ways that assimilate into the local cultures and which are compatible with any local habitus. At a more political level we might be inclined to try to change the culture itself so that youngsters are able to make better informed and more enlightened choices about their lives.

Let us now move away from a focus on young people's sexual health and examine health promotion and communication issues in relation to the more general field of compliance and concordance.

Compliance and concordance

If advice is given, medication dispensed or courses of action agreed upon in a health care consultation, the next step is to wonder whether the directions have been followed. We know from a variety of studies that the level of adherence to the advice or to a recommended treatment regime is often quite low. There are considerable concerns about the impact of poor compliance across a whole range of clinical specialisms and conditions, for example, blood pressure (Bremner 2002), diabetes (Campbell et al. 2003) post-transplant surgery (Chisholm 2002) and mental health (Corriss et al. 1999). Compliance rates are lower where more medication doses have to be taken (Claxton et al. 2001). Sometimes fewer than 50 per cent of patients are believed to be following the optimal course of action with their medication or other therapeutic recommendations. Once lifestyle issues such as diet, smoking and exercise are taken into consideration, rates of compliance with medical advice may be even more disappointing for clinicians.

This issue of whether people comply with courses of treatment is particularly urgent in the UK as there is considerable concern over the national 'drugs bill'. Currently, according to news reports in the UK (Ungoed-Thomas and Templeton 2006) this stands at over £7 billion, for around half a billion prescriptions that are filled annually.

To link these concerns on the part of health care researchers, clinicians and policymakers to something practical and based in communication, let us draw upon some examples of communication in health care consultations where future courses of action were being described from our own research. The examples that follow are from a study of consultations undertaken with nurse advisers by means of the UK's NHS Direct telephone helpline service which we have described in detail elsewhere (Adolphs et al. 2004). Our purpose here is to look at the kinds of linguistic devices used presumably to attempt to secure the caller's interest and commitment to particular courses of action.

First, some overt, quantifiable aspects of the language used by nurse advisers merit our attention, not least the personal pronouns 'you' and 'your'. These occurred significantly more frequently than they do in the English language as a whole and help to secure the hearer's involvement in the consultation. This means that the interactions are very much centred on the caller. The term 'you' was used extensively when giving instructions, identifying courses of action and when advisers used colloquial forms. The following extract illustrates these features:

HA: Yeah, you see you have to do the whole course, you see. Right. What I'm gonna do is just take some details of you for our confidential files.
FP: Eh ha
HA: If I may, and then get a nurse to call you back it will be
FP: OK
HA: Approximately around about 40–45 minutes at the moment.
FP: Or, a little later
HA: ... Thank you very much. Right, have you called us before about yourself?

The focus is thus assiduously upon the client and the client's actions. Intriguingly, there are some asymmetries. The use of 'you' was less intense in the caller's speech, and tended to occur in the phrase 'you know':

> FP: I was just wondering if it could be an allergy should, I mean what should I do, first to get tested obviously I hope, you know phew.

The occasional 'you know' in the caller's discourse is of minor significance by comparison with the overwhelming use of the term in the professionals' language. The frequent use of 'you', even when the callers are not specifically being told to do something, is a feature of persuasive discourse in general and serves to secure the presence of the caller as an object of scrutiny and the subject of future advice. The use of 'you' then is a kind of anchoring device.

Once the involvement and focus in the caller have been secured, it is then the task of the nurse adviser to make the advice appear authoritative. One of the strategies frequently used by the health professionals in these data is the disassociation from the ongoing interaction by either suggesting third-party advice or by referring to secondary sources. In this context it is interesting to note that the lexical item 'able' is used most frequently in the construction 'They'll be able to advise/confirm/look up . . .' Other phrases include 'It says here . . .' or 'The question here is . . .' where the nurse reads out instructions from another source of information. These strategies are mostly successful in that they are rarely challenged by the callers.

To show how the sources of information are deployed in the discourse of the nurse advisers, let us examine a sequence of discourse from the transcribed conversations. Here the caller is concerned with whether it is advisable to drink alcohol while taking antibiotics:

> HA: Here you're there now you're just interested in how much alcohol would be safe to drink with metronbidazeole.
>
> FP: Yeah, yeah
>
> HA: Okay now I've had a look at two sources of information for you. One of them is the British Medical Association their new guide to medicine and drugs.
>
> FP: Eh ha
>
> HA: Now under the alcohol chapter it does suggest that you should avoid it really it said taking with this medication may cause flushing, nausea, vomiting, abdominal pain or headache and I also checked it on the British National Formulary which is a drug interaction checker.
>
> FP: Yeah
>
> HA: And they also said that you'd get a reaction there as well eh so you need to have to be aware if you were to drink then it's probable.
>
> FP: Right
>
> HA: They'll react badly together and sort of give you those symptoms.
>
> FP: Right
>
> HA: And it doesn't really say if there is a safe limit, it's just to avoid altogether really.

In this sequence we can see the sources of authority combined to provide a consolidated prohibition. The individual contributions from the various sources of authority are themselves moralized by the terms used to describe their claims. The BMA guide 'suggests' whereas the BNF says it is 'probable' – both terms are used usually to mitigate the strength of a claim – yet the overall cumulative weight of the recommendations is to 'avoid it altogether'. Indeed, a third source of authority is added later in the interaction:

> HA: You know you could always check with another pharmacist . . .

But the degree of closure imposed by 'altogether' implies that the result of further inquiries would yield the same answer and that they would be redundant – you could ask but you'd get the same answer.

Thus, the credibility of the sources of advice is anchored to concrete items such as books, which are described in some detail – even complementary therapies were anchored to a book called 'medicinal herbs' – which helps to foreground the presence of this authority in the conversation, as if they were actors who speak. The use of sources of authority in book form in this way is rather quaint in some respects, especially in an age of telemedicine when clinicians and researchers themselves are just as likely to use online databases. Nevertheless, it is potent in that it reflects the cultural authority of the written word. Thus, the authority of the advice is established.

Having given advice, the nurses and advisers might well have a stake or interest in whether the caller was at all likely to follow it. Many of the interactions concluded with a sequence which involved a kind of summary of what had been achieved so far so as to encourage the adoption of a course of action. This we called a 'convergence coda' at the end of a stretch of interaction shortly before the phone is put down. For example:

> HA   . . . I certainly learned something by speaking to you tonight. But certainly yeah like I say it may be you know that you might find something helpful.
> FP: Yeah
> HA: In the things I am about to send to you. But if not it's always worthwhile popping them just perhaps to see another GP.
> FP: Yeah
> HA: To see if there is anything else they can do for him, is it OK?
> FP: I'll try that then, great.
> HA: No problem, I'll pop in the post to your work then.
> FP: Lovely
> HA: OK
> FP: Thanks a lot.
> HA: No problem, bye.
> FP: Bye.

In this particular conversation the adviser had addressed the issue of why the caller's husband was getting recurrent earaches and the advisability of seeking a referral for further investigation from his regular GP. In this extract there is a first position invitation to convergence at the suggestion that an opinion from another GP in the practice be sought, yet this yields a 'yeah' rather than an active commitment to do something. The second position invitation – 'To see if there is anything they can do for him, is it OK?'–yields the active agreement to try this approach. Then, the termination sequence can proceed. This kind of termination sequence, where the health adviser, nurse or doctor actively encourages a vocal assent on the part of the client to perform some course of action, may have implications for the study of compliance or concordance.

Of course, the way the debate about concordance and compliance is framed often privileges the view that taking medication as directed is desirable. Incomplete courses of antibiotics are blamed for microbes developing resistance, failure to maintain dosage of a whole variety of treatments for physical and mental health problems is blamed for relapse, and increasing numbers of health problems are seen as resulting from the clients' failure to implement the recommended changes in 'lifestyle': diet, exercise and smoking.

Equally, there may be occasions when people's deviation from treatment regimes occurs on rational grounds that are intelligible to the client and make sense in relation to other debates about the management of one's health. Hopton (2006) gives the example of maintenance medication for schizophrenia associated with, the pervasive professional idea that this 'mental illness' is something that you have to learn to live with, and that only compliance with medication will prevent a relapse. On the other hand, says Hopton, this has medical overtones and is at variance with the view of organizations like the Hearing Voices Network who say that, for some people, hearing voices is merely part of their everyday experience and does not necessarily require 'treatment'. Blaxter and Britten's (1996) review of lay beliefs about medicines explored explanations for the behaviour that professionals find bewildering; they concluded that lay people view medicine as a resource to use as they see fit rather than as something to be taken 'as prescribed'. Pound et al. (2005) note that there may be reasons that are well informed and grounded in experience as to why people do not comply with medication regimes. The side-effects of anti-retroviral regimes for people who are HIV positive, the side-effects from medications for mental health problems, knowledge of adverse drug reactions reported in the press and lay awareness of debates in the professional literature about the desirability of medication may all serve to make people cautious if not actively reluctant to use medication. Thus Pound et al. (2005) use the term 'resistance' to medication. The term resistance was chosen so as to capture lay peoples' 'active engagement with their medicines, as well as the ingenuity and energy they bring to dealing with them. Additionally, it carries the suggestion of something hidden, which is accurate, since most people conceal from their doctors the modifications they make to their regimens' (p. 152).

Thus, once again when we begin to explore the knowledge, habitus and cultural life of participants it makes the apparent failure of communication involved in non-adherence to medical advice appear at once more intelligible and to give the clinician, health educator and policymaker some clues as to how communication may be more readily enhanced.

Conclusions: the cultural situation of health communication

In this chapter we have attempted to review a small part of the literature on communication designed to improve health, promote healthier behaviour and enhance adherence to recommended courses of action. The areas upon which we have concentrated, concerned with smoking, sex, and compliance or concordance have merely scratched the surface of the literature about health communication. However, there are some common themes that run through these three areas which, we would argue, have relevance to other areas of health communication too. That is, we have emphasized the importance of looking at the cultural contexts in which the people targeted by publicity campaigns, advice and medication live and work, and the kinds of knowledge they deploy in their daily lives. We have drawn repeatedly on Bourdieu's notion of 'habitus' to illuminate this. To understand why smoking remains resolutely popular despite half a century of knowledge about its health effects, or why safe sex advice appears to play such a small part in teenagers' romantic engagements, or why people do not take the tablets as directed, we need to understand their habitus. This partly involves understanding what the particular recommended course of action would mean to their social and cultural life. It could place the person in dangerous territory. Being the only smoker in a group of non-smokers, or being a girl who manifestly knows about sex, can place one in a social territory far more immediately threatening than any long-term risk of smoking or unsafe sex itself. Likewise, despite knowledge of appropriate medication adherence, the extent to which one may need to adjust one's life, ignore side-effects and surrender control to the experts may make practical adherence to the medication regime untenable.

This chapter then has tried to examine how what we know about culture and communication might explain why health education based largely on 'information' has only ever had limited success. In order to make progress here, perhaps we should reconceptualize the role of the communicator as that of the anthropologist. Knowledge of the culture and social practices of the participants concerned might well be helpful in designing interventions. At the very least, it must be explored as an alternative to simply wringing our hands at clients' lack of knowledge or their apparent inability to follow simple instructions. These are not merely lapses or deficiencies, we would suggest, but might represent aspects of a culture which, as Pound et al. (2005) suggest, are often hidden from health professionals.

References

Adolphs, S., Brown, B., Carter, R., Crawford, P. and Sahota, O. (2004) Applying corpus linguistics in a health care context, *Journal of Applied Linguistics*, 1(1): 9–28.

Amos, A., Wiltshire, S., Bostock, Y., Haw, S. and McNeill, A. (2004) 'You can't go without a fag ... you need it for your hash': a qualitative exploration of smoking, cannabis and young people, *Addiction*, 99: 77–81.

Bandura, A. (1977) *Social Learning Theory*. Englewood Cliffs, NJ: Prentice Hall.

Bartky, S.L. (1990) *Femininity and Domination: Studies in the Phenomenology of Domination*. London: Routledge.

Beck, U. (1992) *Risk Society: Towards a New Modernity*. London: Sage.

Blaxter, M. and Britten, N. (1996) *Lay Beliefs about Drugs and Medicines and the Implications for Pharmacy*. Manchester: Pharmacy Practice Research Resource Centre.

Blum, R.W., Beuhring, T., Wunderlich, M. and Resnick, M.D. (1996) Don't ask, they won't tell: the quality of adolescent health screening in five practice settings, *American Journal of Public Health*, 86: 1767–72.

Boreham, R. and Shaw, A. (2001) *Smoking Drinking and Drug Use in Scotland in 2000*. Edinburgh: Stationery Office.

Bourdieu, P. (1984) *Distinction: A Social Critique of the Judgment of Taste*. Cambridge, MA: Harvard University Press.

Bourdieu, P. (1990) *The Logic of Practice*. Stanford, CA: Stanford University Press.

Bremner, A.D. (2002) Antihypertensive medication and quality of life: silent treatment of a silent killer, *Cardiovascular Drugs and Therapy*, 16: 353–64.

British Lung Foundation (2002) *A Smoking Gun: The Impact of Cannabis Smoking on Respiratory Health*. London: British Lung Foundation.

Brook Advisory Centres (2002) *Teenage Sexual Activity. Factsheet 1, April*. London: Brook Advisory Centres.

Burrack, R. (1999) Teenage sexual behaviour: attitudes towards and declared sexual activity, *British Journal of Family Planning*, 24: 145–8.

Campbell, R., Pound, P., Pope, C. et al. (2003) Evaluating meta ethnography: a synthesis of qualitative research on lay experiences of diabetes and diabetes care, *Social Science and Medicine*, 56(4): 671–84.

Cancer Research UK (2005) *Lung Cancer Factsheet*. Available at http://info.cancerresearch-uk.org/images/publicationspdfs/factsheet_lung_cancer.pdf (accessed 19 March 2006).

Chassin, L., Presson, C.C., Sherman, S.J. and Pitts, S.C. (2000) The natural history of cigarette smoking from adolescence to adulthood in a Midwestern community sample: Multiple trajectories and their psychosocial correlates, *Health Psychology*, 19: 223–31.

Chisholm, M. (2002) Enhancing transplant patients' adherence to medication therapy, *Clinical Transplantation*, 16: 30–8.

Clark, H.W., Horton, A.M., Dennis, M. and Babor, T.F. (2002) Moving from research to practice just in time: the treatment of cannabis use comes of age, *Addiction*, 97 (suppl.): s1–s3.

Claxton, A.J., Cramer, J. and Pierce, C. (2001) A systematic review of the relationship between dose regimens and medication compliance, *Clinical Therapeutics*, 23(8): 1296–310.

Cohen, P. and Ainley, P. (2000) In the country of the blind? Youth studies and cultural studies in Britain, *Journal of Youth Studies*, 3(1): 79–95.

Connell, P., McKevitt, C. and Low, N. (2004) Investigating ethnic differences in sexual health: focus groups with young people, *Sexually Transmitted Infections*, 80: 300–5.

Corriss, D.J., Smith, T.E., Hull, J.W., Lim, R.W., Pratt, S.I. and Romanelli, S. (1999) Interactive risk factors for treatment adherence in a chronic psychotic disorders population, *Psychiatry Research*, 89: 269–74.

Cowie, C. and Lees, S. (1987) Slags and drags, in Feminist Review (eds) *Sexuality: A Reader*. London: Virago.

De Gaston, J.F., Weed, S. and Jensen, L. (1996) Understanding gender differences in adolescent sexuality, *Adolescence*, 31: 217–31.

Dicenso, A., Guyatt, G., Willan, A. and Griffith, L. (2002) Interventions to reduce unintended pregnancies among adolescents: systematic review of randomized controlled trials, *British Medical Journal*, 324: 1426–33.

Doll, R. and Hill, A.B. (1950) Smoking and carcinoma of the lung: Preliminary report, *British Medical Journal*, 2: 739–48.

Drummond, C. (2002) Cannabis control: costs outweigh the benefits – against, *British Medical Journal*, 342: 106–8.

Ellickson, P.L., Tucker, J.S. and Klein, D.J. (2001) High-risk behaviors associated with early smoking: results from a 5-year follow-up, *Journal of Adolescent Health*, 28: 465–73.

Escobedo, L.G., Reddy, M. and DuRant, R.H. (1997) Relationship between cigarette smoking and health risk and problem behaviors among US adolescents, *Archives of Pediatric and Adolescent Medicine*, 151: 66–71.

Evans, D.L. and Tripp, J.H. (2006) Sex education: the case for primary prevention and peer education, *Current Paediatrics*, 16: 95–9.

Exner, M. (1915) Sex education by the Young Men's Christian Association in universities and colleges, *Journal of Social Hygiene*, 1(4): 570–80.

Ford, D.E., Vu, H.T. and Anthony, J.C. (2002) Marijuana use and cessation of tobacco smoking in adults from a community sample, *Drug and Alcohol Dependence*, 67: 243–8.

Foucault, M. (1977) *Discipline and Punish: The Birth of the Prison* (translated by A. Sheridan). Harmondsworth: Penguin.

Fraser, F. (2002) *Drug Misuse in Scotland: Findings from the 2000 Scottish Crime Survey*. Edinburgh: Scottish Executive Central Research Unit.

Frederick, K. and Barlow, J. (2006) The Citizenship Safety Project: a pilot study, *Health Education Research*, 21(1): 87–96.

Gabriel, S.J. and Todorova, E.O. (2003) Racism and capitalist accumulation: an overdetermined nexus, *Critical Sociology*, 29(1): 29–46.

Goold, P.C., Bustard, S., Ferguson, E., Carlin, E.M., Neal, K. and Bowman, C.A. (2006) Pilot study in the development of an Interactive Multimedia Learning Environment for sexual health interventions: a focus group approach, *Health Education Research*, 21(1): 15–25.

Health Protection Agency (2003) *Renewing the Focus: HIV and other Sexually Transmitted Infections in the United Kingdom in 2002*. London: Health Protection Agency.

Heath, S. (1982) *The Sexual Fix*. Basingstoke: Macmillan.

Henry, J.A., Oldfield, W.L.G. and Kon, O.M. (2003) Comparing cannabis with tobacco, *British Medical Journal*, 326: 942–3.

Holland, J., Ramzanoglu, C., Sharpe, S. and Thomas, R. (1996) Reputations: journeying into gendered power relations, in J. Weeks and J. Holland (eds) *Sexual Cultures, Communities, Values and Intimacy*. London: Macmillan.

Hopton, J. (2006) The future of critical psychiatry, *Critical Social Policy*, 26(1): 57–73.

Hyde, A., Howlett, E., Drennan, J. and Brady, D. (2005) Masculinities and young men's sex education needs in Ireland: problematizing client-centred health promotion approaches, *Health Promotion International*, 20(4): 334–41.

Johnson, P.B. and Richter, L. (2002) The relationship between smoking, drinking, and adolescents' self-perceived health and frequency of hospitalization: analyses from the

1997 National Household Survey on Drug Abuse, *Journal of Adolescent Health*, 30: 175–83.

Johnston, L.D., O'Malley, P.M. and Bachman, J.G. (2003) *Monitoring the Future. National Results on Adolescent Drug Use: Overview of Key Findings 2002* (NIH Publication No. 03–5374). Bethesda, MD: National Institute on Drug Abuse.

Kitzinger, J. (1995) 'I'm sexually attractive but I'm powerful': young women negotiating sexual reputation, *Women's Studies International Forum*, 18(2): 187–96.

Lawy, R. (2002) Risky stories: youth identities, learning and everyday risk, *Journal of Youth Studies*, 5(4): 407–23.

Lees, S. (1993) *Sugar and Spice: Sexuality and Adolescent Girls*. London: Penguin.

Lucas, K. and Lloyd, B. (1999) Starting smoking: girls' explanations of the influence of peers, *Journal of Adolescence*, 22: 647–55.

McGuire, W.J. (1969) The nature of attitudes and attitude change, in G. Lindzey and E. Aronson (eds) *Handbook of Social Psychology*, Vol. 3. Reading, MA: Addison-Wesley.

Mason, L. (2005) 'They haven't a clue!' A qualitative study of staff perceptions of 11–14-year-old female clinic attenders, *Primary Health Care Research and Development*, 6: 199–207.

Maton, K. (2003) Reflexivity, relationism, and research: Pierre Bourdieu and the epistemic conditions of social scientific knowledge, *Space and Culture*, 6: 52–65.

Mouffe, C. (2005) *On the Political*. London: Routledge.

Office for National Statistics (2003) *Living in Britain: General Household Survey 2003*. London: Office for National Statistics.

Office for National Statistics (2004) *Smoking Related Behaviour and Attitudes 2003*. London: Office for National Statistics.

OFSTED (2002) *Sex and Relationships*. London: OFSTED.

Orlando, M., Tucker, J.S., Ellickson, P.L. and Klein, D.J. (2004) Developmental trajectories of cigarette smoking and their correlates from early adolescence to young adulthood, *Journal of Consulting and Clinical Psychology*, 72: 400–10.

Parker, H., Williams, L. and Aldridge, J. (2002) The normalization of 'sensible' drug use: further evidence from the North England Longitudinal Study, *Sociology*, 36(4): 941–64.

Pitts, M., Burtney, E. and Dobraszczyc, U. (1996) 'There is no shame in it any more': how providers of sexual health advice view young people's sexuality, *Health Education Research: Theory and Practice*, 11: 1–9.

Plumridge, E.W., Fitzgerald, L.J. and Abel, G.M. (2002) Performing coolness: smoking refusal and adolescent identities, *Health Education Research: Theory and Practice*, 17(2): 167–79.

Poland, B., Frohlich, K., Haines, R.J., Mykhalovskiy, E., Rock, M. and Sparks, R. (2006) The social context of smoking: the next frontier in tobacco control? *Tobacco Control*, 15: 59–63.

Porter, C.P. (2002) Female 'tweens' and sexual development, *Journal of Paediatric Nursing*, 17: 402–6.

Potts, A. (2002) *The Science/Fiction of Sex: Feminist Deconstruction and the Vocabularies of Heterosex*. London: Routledge.

Poulin, C. and Graham, L. (2001) The association between substance use, unplanned sexual intercourse and other sexual behaviours among adolescent students, *Addiction*, 96: 607–21.

Pound, P., Britten, N., Morgan, M. et al. (2005) Resisting medicines: a synthesis of qualitative studies of medicine taking, *Social Science and Medicine*, 61: 133–55.

Prince, F. (1995) The relative effectiveness of a peer-led and adult-led smoking intervention
programme, *Adolescence*, 30: 187–94.

Ramsay, G. (1943) The sex information of younger boys, *American Journal of Orthopsychiatry*,
13: 34–43.

Rogers, E.M. (1983) *Diffusion of Innovations*, 3rd edn. New York: The Free Press.

Ruch, G. (2002) From triangle to spiral: reflective practice in social work education, practice
and research, *Social Work Education*, 21: 199–216.

Schofield, M. (1973) *The Sexual Behaviour of Young Adults*. London: Allen Lane.

Social Exclusion Unit (1992) *Teenage Pregnancy*. London: Stationery Office.

Stewart, F. (1999) 'Once you get a reputation, your life's like . . . wrecked': The implication of
reputation for young women's sexual health and well-being, *Women's Studies International Forum*, 22(3): 373–83.

Substance Abuse and Mental Health Services Administration (SAMHSA) (2003) *Overview of
Findings from the 2002 National Survey on Drug Use and Health (Office of Applied Studies,
NHSDA Series H-21*, DHHS Publication No. SMA 03–3774). Rockville, MD: SAMHSA.

Svenson, G.R. (1998) *European Guidelines for Youth AIDS Peer Education in Sweden*. Lund:
European Commission.

Tucker, J.S., Ellickson, P.A., Orlando, M. and Klein, D.J. (2006) Cigarette smoking from
adolescence to young adulthood: women's developmental trajectories and associated
outcomes, *Women's Health Issues*, 16: 30–7.

Ungoed-Thomas, J. and Templeton, S.-K. (2006) Nurses earn bonuses for the use of latest
drugs, *Sunday Times*, 5 March.

US Department of Health and Human Services (USDHHS) (2001) *Women and Smoking: A
Report of the Surgeon General*. Rockville, MD: USDHHS, PHS, Office of the Surgeon
General.

von Glasersfeld, E. (1991) Knowing without metaphysics: aspects of the radical con-
structivist position, in F. Steier (ed.) *Research and Reflexivity*. London: Sage.

Walker, B. (1997) 'You learn it from your mates don't you?' Young people's conversations as
a basis for informal peer education, *Youth and Policy*, 57: 44–54.

Walker, J., MacGillivray, I. and MacNaughton, M. (eds) (1976) *Combined Textbook of
Obstetrics and Gynaecology*, 9th edn. Edinburgh: Churchill Livingstone.

White, D. and Pitts, M. (1997) *Health Promotion in Young People for the Prevention of Substance
Misuse*. London: Health Education Authority.

Wight, D., Henderson, M., Raab, G. et al. (2000) Extent of regretted sexual intercourse
among young teenagers in Scotland: a cross sectional survey, *British Medical Journal*,
320: 1243–4.

Wilson, H. and Huntington, A. (2005) Deviant (m)others: the construction of teenage
motherhood in contemporary discourse, *Journal of Social Policy*, 35(1): 59–76.

10 Blip culture: the power of brief communication

Fast health care

Over a quarter of a century ago Alvin Toffler envisioned a future characterized by what he called 'blip culture'. In this, 'instead of receiving long, related "strings" of ideas, organized or synthesized for us, we are increasingly exposed to short, modular blips of information – adverts, commands, theories, shreds of news … that refuse to fit neatly into our pre-existing mental files' (1980: 182). In the same way, a great many health care encounters are taking place in short 'blips' often of five minutes or less across a range of sites and involving a vast number of practitioners. From acute admissions wards to nursing homes, from scanner suites to complementary practitioners, NHS walk-in centres to plastic surgeons, the public encounter a variety of fragments of health care communication. As we outlined earlier, what is needed is a comprehensive model of how all these brief encounters can be part of the therapeutic milieu.

This chapter will aim to distil from existing literature and our own research a way of understanding health care encounters of five minutes or less, and emphasize how even momentary communications can convey support, warmth and a sense of inclusion. We will write about pragmatic communication as much as evidence-based communication. This would have impact on communication teaching skills since currently counselling models dominate. Yet the latter often conflict with practice realities. We require a new paradigm for communication skills teaching that enhances skills at delivering high quality engagement in the briefest time. For example, it should be possible to communicate even in passing in a corridor or on a ward and provide comfort and support on the hoof. The skill element in communication might be more to do with strategies for identifying and responding to opportunities for interaction – so successful health care communicators may be those who adapt to task-dominated environments and utilize even momentary time slots to good effect. This backcloth of successive momentary engagement and warmth could create a positive realm for recovery.

There is a great deal of literature which emphasizes the importance and value of good interpersonal relations between clients and professionals in health care, yet a major issue facing health care professionals is that of finding time for communication with clients. In an era when many practice areas, clinics and teams are increasingly task driven and concerned to boost their productivity, communication can actually slow down the 'people processing'. There is a sense then that communication can 'get in the way' of health care encounters. There are a great many situations where punctuality is at a premium and time is of the essence. Getting nursing home residents ready for bed, administering injections or weighing infants can all be performed more speedily if communication is kept to a minimum. From the clients' point of view this is often most unsatisfactory and can lead to a sense of alienation and complaints that care is perfunctory or inhumane. Indeed, where clients are confused or require reassurance it might even lead to violence. Thus, the organizational constraints tend to press staff ever more firmly towards brevity, yet most interpersonal models of care tend to emphasize aspects of the process which require time for interaction and mutual storytelling. In practical contexts communication is often targeted rather than utilizing discursive approaches. To date, interpersonal philosophies and frameworks of care have avoided time consciousness as a key issue, and instead tend to promote more extended forms of communication based around notions of therapeutic relationships, deepening empathy, mutual understanding and regard for clients.

A 1998 survey of 302 UK GPs reported that 'the major perceived barrier to practising evidence-based medicine was lack of personal time' (McColl et al. 1998: 361). In a 1999 study of eight UK NHS general practices, the most commonly referred to concern relating to the practice environment was lack of time, and the study noted that the strength of feeling about this was considerable. Lack of time was seen as hindering effectiveness in many aspects of medical practice (Tomlin et al. 1999). A 1999/2000 survey of Australian GPs (Young and Ward 2001: 205) reported that lack of time was rated as a 'very important barrier' to searching for and appraising evidence, and to discussing the implications of evidence with patients.

As Christakis and Feudtner put it:

> Although most patients may perceive a 2-minute encounter with a physician seated at the bedside as more reassuring then a 2-minute chat with him standing at the doorjamb 2 minutes is still only 2 minutes; patients placated enough to comply (or not complain), still may not feel connected to their physicians in any meaningful sense ... The healing touch in major medical centers rarely lingers. Patients suffer – and so too do those who desire to be healers ... A student or house officer may wonder, 'would it be right for me, a temporary stranger, who just wandered into these patients' lives, to engage them on an intimate level when I only spend 8 hours on call with them? Wouldn't that be the emotional or therapeutic equivalent of a one-night stand?' We believe that too many students and residents incur long-term personal damage by engaging in transient relationships with strangers.
>
> (1997: 742)

The impetus for considering brief communication in health care communication comes from several sources. Our observations of communication in health care have suggested a curious contradiction. The brief kinds of jolly, supportive or encouraging communication that we use in everyday life with friends and family often disappear in clinical sites. In other words, professionals seem to adopt formal, neutralized expressions in preference to ordinary and emotionally generous remarks or gestures. Sometimes, whereas the briefest of conversations with a friend can leave one with a good and lasting feeling of self-worth, the kinds of neglectful, perfunctory or unemotional exchanges in clinical sites can leave clients or patients feeling profoundly isolated and ignored. The transformational strengths of kind, ordinary and friendly exchanges appear overlooked in health care. Traditionally, health communication curricula have focused on teaching counselling and processing skills – the former welded to professionalism and expertise; the latter to business and economic efficiency. But the simpler, briefer interactions, for example, a smile with the aura of authenticity rather than the gloss of one encouraged by 'customer care' training, are demoted as taken for granted. In this chapter we are intending to explore some of what is missing from many clinical encounters, and explore some means of thinking about or theorizing this element, by considering a number of traditions of work in anthropology, linguistics and sociology which have tried to get a grip on what happens in conversation to generate this immediate sense of warmth. This will equip us to explore in finer detail how this inconsistency comes about between personal and professional styles of communication, and how we can enable health professionals to make the best use of the few moments of consultation time they may have. Health professionals are increasingly called upon to demonstrate the effectiveness not only of specific interventions but of their role as a whole (Irvine-Doran et al. 2002). The practitioners are often perfectly capable of making friends and family members feel good from a very brief interaction. Yet in Kasper's (1992: 2) words, they 'don't always use what they know' in professional contexts.

An important source of insight in this area concerns the variety of literatures about how mood and emotion are related to communication. Ethnographic, anthropological and linguistic accounts of communicative features such as greetings or compliments underline the role they play in cementing positive social bonds. There is also a strand of scholarship in speech act theory which stresses what people do with words and how in some cases language is performative rather than merely descriptive. The phrase 'How do you do?', for example, is not necessarily a question but instead is often part of a symbolic greeting sequence and so does not demand a literal or detailed answer. In some ethnolinguistic communities the phrase 'Where are you going?' performs much the same function.

Phatic communication and the language of face work

Related to this, there is another tradition in anthropology and linguistics involving the study of so called 'phatic' communication. The idea of phatic communication was first popularized by the anthropologist Malinowski (1922) who used the term to refer to 'language used in free, aimless, social intercourse'. Brown and Levinson (1987) note that 'the subject of talk is not as important as the fact of carrying on a conversation that is amply loaded with ... markers of emotional agreement'. Some thinkers in health care such as Burnard (2003) have begun to consider the role of these processes in health care communication. Burnard provides some extracts which distinguish between the more businesslike and more phatic kinds of communication. A businesslike exchange might take a form like the following:

Nurse: Good morning
Patient: Morning
Nurse: I want to take your blood pressure please.
Patient: OK, thank you.

(p. 680)

Here, the use of a more formal greeting serves as an indicator to the patient that the exchange is likely to be a businesslike one – as indeed it turns out. A phatic exchange might resemble the following:

Nurse: Hello, Mrs. Jones, how are you?
Patient: I'm not too bad, thank you, despite things really . . .
Nurse: You don't sound too sure!
Patient: Well, those new tablets are making me feel awful.
Nurse: Which ones?
Patient: The antidepressants. They are upsetting my stomach.
Nurse: Are you sure it is those ones that are doing it?
Patient: Yes, the doctor took me off the other ones and these ones are giving me a terrible stomach.
Nurse: OK, well we need to do something about that . . .

(pp. 680–1)

Here, an excursion into phatic metacommentary on the emotional tone of the conversation 'you don't sound too sure' elicits a piece of potentially useful information. These kinds of departures from the formal protocol are quickly and easily accomplished yet can be very useful in eliciting information and tailoring the delivery of care to the clients' needs.

Coupland et al. (1992) note that phatic communications may be used strategically so as to secure the cooperation of the other parties to the interaction, and Jefferson (1984) notes that laughter can be used in troubles talk so as to demonstrate a mutually agreeable resistance to troubles. Similarly, much of the laughter detectable in conversation is an orderly, consequential action and can be used to increase the sense of intimacy between interactants (Jefferson et al. 1987). As Boyle (2000) argues, appropriately timed laughter can be used to signal affiliation between the participants in a conversation.

Coupland et al. (1992) describe phatic communion as involving apparent aimlessness but on the other hand might at the same time be fulfilling important functions: 'talk that is aimless, prefatory, obvious, uninteresting, sometimes suspect, and even irrelevant, but part of the process of fulfilling our intrinsically human needs for social cohesiveness and mutual recognition' (p. 209). Such everyday matters as greetings and goodbyes, thanks and compliments are aspects of phatic communion that enhance social cohesion. Laver (1975, 1981) argues that the phatic function of actions such as compliments is a 'propitiatory' or emollient one. To make small talk or extend greeting exchanges defuses 'the potential hostility of silence in situations where speech is conventionally anticipated' (1981: 301).

As Boyle (2000) notes, another important phatic function is an exploratory one, which 'carries the conversational implicature of negotiating a change in the relationship between the participants, usually towards greater intimacy or greater distancing' (Laver 1981: 304). In this exploratory role, phatic communication has an inherent and valuable ambiguity which allows it to be used dissimulatively.

On the other hand if we take the perspective of Garfinkel (1967) and Boyle (2000), this idea that phatic communication can get important work done makes sense.

As Bolton (2001) describes it, examples of humorous or lighthearted communication in a hospital setting can have a very valuable function even when they are transitory or trivial. Often in discussing life in health care settings authors and practitioners have focused on the tragic or sorrowful aspects of the situation. Yet there are various ways in which practitioners can, however fleetingly, offer what Bolton calls a 'gift' of communication that is based around fun or pleasure. Bolton describes how nurses frequently offer humour as a means of 'getting through'. Humour may reflect the pleasure practitioners gain from interaction with patients and with one another (Fox 1990). Nurses may introduce humour into their work as a way of easing tension or embarrassment, or because, as one of Bolton's (2001) informants put it: 'the place needed lightening'. Having used humour in this way practitioners report feeling immediately rewarded with the sense of wellbeing this creates on the ward. One particular ward sister was described as pushing the medication trolley shouting 'ice-creams, sweeties' and would stand in the middle of the ward and entertain the patients and her colleagues with anecdotes about herself and her husband, and how her husband has taken to calling her 'my little swamp duck'. Bolton discovered when speaking to patients who have been on this ward that they remember this particular sister with fondness and in some cases attributed their successful recovery to having a 'good laugh'.

These kinds of manoeuvres can be linked to the notion of the 'recipient design' of turns in conversation (Sacks et al. 1974: 727). This was identified as a pervasive tendency in ordinary conversation which particularizes conversational interaction and matches it to the needs of the hearer. As Sacks et al. (1974: 727) put it: 'By "recipient design" we refer to a multitude of respects in which the talk by a party in a conversation is constructed or designed in ways which display an orientation and sensitivity to the particular other(s) who are the co-participants'.

In this way the basics of greeting and extracting information and applying interventions can be more effectively tailored to clients' needs. This is especially so if practitioners are empowered to follow up intuitions about the mood or demeanour of the client. This need not be drawn out over a whole consultation, but can be incorporated into incidental remarks and casual interaction.

A further strand of scholarship that has some relevance to the issue here is symbolic interactionism and Goffman's (1955) concept of 'face' and 'face work'. The concept of *face* is generally understood in sociology and linguistics as 'the negotiated public image, mutually granted each other by participants in a communicative event', and it is located in the very flow of our daily communication (Scollon and Scollon 1995). It is the 'positive social value' that individuals want to create and/or maintain to themselves (Goffman 1955: 213). The idea of being able to maintain positive 'face' might be particularly important in health care contexts where examinations and interventions might well be painful or humiliating. Thus, an examination of the face-threatening elements of a clinical encounter and how they might be mitigated may well be extremely valuable in health care contexts. In Goffman's (1967: 19) words, 'one's face is a sacred thing, and the expressive order required to sustain it is therefore a ritual one'. The self is 'a ritually delicate object' (p. 31). 'When a face has been threatened, facework must be done' (p. 27).

For example, Bolton (2001) has documented the kinds of strategies which experienced nurses see themselves as using to manage the emotional content of their working lives. There is a sense even among experienced nurses that they could or should do more:

> I went home the other night thinking I could have been kinder to Mr. So and So. After all he is really worried about his wife and it's not up to him to know what sort of day it had been. But it was all I could do to present him with the facts in a calm, empty sort of way. I was on the brink of bawling myself, we'd had eight miscarriages and two deaths and I was worn out with it all. But I feel really sorry now that he didn't get what he should have got. I'm sure he'll be back. I suspect his wife is in for a run, so I'll try to make it up another time (senior staff nurse).
>
> (p. 92)

Strauss et al. (1982: 254) were among the first to coin the phrase, 'sentimental work', in recognition that 'there is more to medical work than its physiological core'. At the same time, the sentimental encounter is not one between equals but is frequently structured in dominance. Power is often seen as a central factor in encounters between professionals and clients, and research within a power framework was oriented to demonstrate how clients had 'smaller and less significant space on the linguistic floor' than professionals (Brown et al. 1996). Yet at the same time there is evidence that patients want more. In Shattrell's (2004) work patients longed for more and deeper connections with nurses. They experienced the hospital environment as disconnecting and actively sought ways to connect with nurses. Patients' dependence on nursing staff as well as perceived powerlessness in relation to the nurse's power, created a situation where patients believed they had 'actively' to find ways to solicit the nursing care they needed.

There is clearly a good deal more going on here than the meaning of the words if one looked them up in a dictionary. All these functions of language would only be partially addressed if we focused solely on the meaning of the terms in the conversation. What we are driving at is that to make sense of communication in health care we need to grasp the pragmatic functions of language, smiles, humour and gesture. In pragmatics attention is devoted to the way in which context influences the meaning and interpretation of language by the speakers and hearers. Competence in pragmatics, however, is 'a delicate area and it is not immediately obvious how it can be "taught"' (Bou-Franch and Garces-Conejos 2003).

Lakoff (1989: 102–3) states that ordinary conversation functions as a template for other forms of interaction 'which we experience in terms of their similarities to and differences from ordinary conversation and feel more or less comfortable with to the degree that they conform to our ordinary-conversation-based expectations'.

Developing skills in conversational pragmatics and in implementing what they know about how to hold a conversation outside the clinical context may well improve practitioners' work with clients. In second-language acquisition, educators and theorists often talk about developing in the student some 'metapragmatic ability', which involves 'the ability to analyse language use in a conscious manner' (Thomas 1983: 98).

In essence, an evidence-based focus on brief communication may break the log-jam of traditional counselling approaches in health curricula that skew towards mental health contexts. It would promote quick, generic and pragmatic communication along an axis of skilled ordinariness (Carter 2004). As Burnard (2003: 682) puts it, when talking about mental health nurses: '[they] may be remembered as much for their friendliness and ordinariness as for their counseling skills. Ordinary chat might be as important as therapeutic conversation'.

This opens up a number of possibilities. For example, some styles of communication are a kind of time management. Closing a consultation may be expedited by gestures like closing the file. In order to achieve rapid, effective and emotionally supportive communications, practitioners need a reality-driven conception of communicative practice. At present a good deal of training is driven by an implicit model that sees counselling as the ideal to which practitioners should aspire. However, in practice settings task-focused communication that conveys meanings in a minimal or economic way is the target.

Therefore, to make sense of the brevity of many health care encounters and draw on the kinds of communicative expertise professionals and clients display to offer recommendations for practice we need a way of extracting the best elements from 'time-generous' philosophies of communication and applying them to 'time-sensitive' settings of the kind in which health care is often practised.

Making sense of how a whole emotional lexicon of feelings and ideas might be communicated in relatively short health care encounters involves us in retheorizing communication in health care in a way that does not demonize professionals or see lack of communication as a deficiency in skills. Instead we want to develop a new conception of health care communication along the lines of what can realistically be achieved in demanding situations.

Emotional tone and emotion work: the labours of love

In brief encounters in health care settings, while there may be limited opportunities for extensive information exchange, the relatively fleeting interactions may contain ample opportunities for emotional tone to be conveyed. For example tired, dour expressions and lacklustre demeanour, combined with monosyllabic, grumpily delivered speech communicate a message of misery in a matter of seconds. The effects of emotions and moods on organizational behaviour in health care settings can be complex and varied, in line with participants' socio-cognitive constructions of their emotional situations.

When the interactional encounters in a workplace setting have to involve a particular kind of emotional tone, the term 'emotional labour' is sometimes used to describe an important aspect of the work they involve. The concept of emotional labour was first promoted by Hochschild, in a study of cabin crew on aircraft, who had to maintain polite and pleasant contact with passengers and keep smiling even on long and arduous flights. She noted that emotions were displayed according to a 'set of shared, albeit often latent, rules' (1983: 268) which governed the kinds of emotions which were specific to each situation. The parallels with the work situation of health care practitioners were quickly noted (Bolton 2001; Mann and Cowburn 2005). Emotional labour, across a whole range of service industries, has been described as the effort involved when employees 'regulate their emotional display in an attempt to meet organizationally based expectations specific to their roles' (Brotheridge and Lee 2003: 365). It is also closely related to Strauss et al.'s (1982: 254) 'sentimental work', a concept introduced to help explore the possibility that 'there was more to medical work than its physiological core'. While Strauss et al. (1982) compare 'sentimental work' to tender loving care they also point out that it is performed as a means of getting the 'work done effectively' rather than exclusively out of humane concerns.

Emotion work is closely allied to the idea that there are 'display rules' or 'expectations' governing the kinds of emotions that can be expressed and how they may be exhibited. These may specify, either formally or informally, which emotions employees ought to express and which ought to be suppressed. Practitioners may want to portray emotions in accordance with display rules because they care about their clients, or keeping their jobs, or because there are occasions when genuinely felt emotions do not concur with those it is judged appropriate to display. Feeling one thing and displaying another is at the very heart of emotional labour.

As well as displaying certain emotions, emotional labour involves controlling others. Emotional labour strategically allows practitioners to present an impersonal approach to colleagues, clients and society as a whole, especially when dealing with difficult moments such as death and dying (Sudnow 1967), mistakes (Bosk 1979), and with the uncertainties inevitably involved in trying to apply medical knowledge (Fox 1980).

Often, there is a sense of trying to fit one's emotions to those of the client one is dealing with at the time. A nurse in Staden's (1998: 152–3) study said that when working with a depressed or distressed patient, 'even if you may be feeling quite buoyant yourself, you will dampen down ... the image you portray on your face ... so that it matches ... the mood'.

Emotion work, like the phatic communication we described earlier, could be deployed strategically to achieve therapeutic ends. A nurse's caring skills are in a sense a political instrument as they may be used as a resource to manipulate the image of health care in order to achieve financial (Phillips 1996), or 'socio-cultural and wider political ends' (O'Brien 1994: 393). Yet emotion work in health care settings is not exclusively about an economically motivated process of exchange. As Bolton (2001) argues, as social beings, emotion management by health care practitioners is a way of 'paying respect with feeling'; it is a personal gift given freely, sometimes unconsciously, and sometimes without the counting of costs, and as Mann and Cowburn (2005) add, many practitioners felt that their emotional labour performance helped the clients cope with their own emotions. Indeed, Bolton (2001: 86) described nurses as 'accomplished social actors and multiskilled emotion managers'.

Brief encounters: health care and the comfort of strangers

The fleeting and transient encounters between strangers that are characteristic of the delivery of health care in the UK seem set to become even more widespread. Rather than a longstanding relationship with a GP, ever larger numbers of patients will be seen by a variety of professionals employed by group practices and primary care trusts. In the UK there are also telephone helplines, walk-in centres and a variety of outreach services for sex workers, rough sleepers and other marginalized groups, all of which are supplementing the traditional primary care arrangements. The NHS itself claims that 5 million patients have used its growing numbers of walk-in centres, and at the time of writing, more are opening, especially at railway stations (NHS Direct 2006).

The brevity of encounters between practitioners and clients who have had little or no prior relationship are perhaps also best placed in context against the growing rate of migration between nations. This further reduces the opportunities for longer term supportive relationships to develop between health care providers and clients and highlights the necessity for effective brief communication that can reach across language or cultural divisions. Presently it is estimated that 8 per cent of the European population and 11.5 per cent of the US population could be classified as migrants (Global Commission on International Migration 2004).

Let us return to the issue of sexual health by way of an illustration. Serrant-Green (2005) notes that research into problems identified by minority ethnic participants accessing sexual health services suggests the desirability of a greater focus on general issues relating to the lifestyles of ethnic minorities. There are a number of aspects of communication between practitioners and transient or socially marginal clients that clients feel are important yet do not necessarily take long to establish. Here are some participants in a study by McCoy of the experience of being HIV positive discussing what they find desirable in their relationship with their doctors.

> Participant 1: It is a trust thing. I do not mean I want to get personal with them, I just want to feel that they are not aloof, they are not above me, they are not better than I am.
>
> Participant 2: For me it is comfort level. That is, you know, to have a relationship with the doctor is that I have the comfort level that I feel that I can ask or scream in his or her face if I feel I need to and that is going to be accepted as OK – not that I do. That if I really feel strongly about something that I can say it. A respect. (FG 11)
>
> (2005: 798)

These speakers, from socially marginalized communities in Canada, were particularly concerned with the quality of relationship they perceived they had with their doctors. Issues such as 'trust' and 'respect' were described as desirable. In McCoy's study some participants talked about trusting the doctor's expertise or motives, but here trust also seems to connote the ideas they had about expectations of the doctor's possible response to the issues they raise: it refers to their belief that the doctor will not 'brush them off' or belittle them. In the second quotation, the speaker makes a similar point and describes the key element as 'a respect' which, if it is evinced by the doctor, makes him feel comfortable, and the sense of disapproval which has accrued from many authority figures in the past will be less stultifying. McCoy (2005: 798) believes that in this context respect is the 'flip side' of trust: 'trust is what patients feel and do when doctors feel and express respect'.

Now, from the point of view of our interest in brief communication, what is interesting here is that the first participant links his ability to 'trust' to the practitioner not acting 'aloof' or superior. Perhaps the interactional sense of solidarity and reduction of social distance is a component of this sense of respect. From McCoy's account it seems to be something that can be cultivated relatively quickly. In terms of Brown and Levinson's (1987:62) notion of 'politeness' it creates a sense of involvement or belonging in a group, which addresses the desire to be 'ratified, understood, approved of, liked or admired'.

'Time tardises' and indexicality

Managing limited time and ensuring that the patients or clients get the best out of the encounter, no matter how brief, is essential. One idea, which is all the more interesting because it intersects neatly with a key concept from ethnomethodology, is that of the 'time tardis'. The concept is not our own, but originates with an Australasian colleague, Wendy Hu. Like the tardis in the popular science fiction series, *Dr Who*, the encounter needs to be bigger 'inside' than it looks from the 'outside'. Part of this process involves 'housekeeping factors' such as whether the phone can be prevented from ringing and whether colleagues can be prevented from interrupting, so as to create a sense that one is focusing on the client.

Some clinicians with resources and assistants at their command can use two consulting rooms so that an assistant can 'greet and seat' the client in one room while the practitioner is finishing off the previous consultation in the other, and then stride into the room and begin the consultation immediately, while the assistant is showing the previous client out and the next one in. This is described as minimizing the 'dead time'. On the other hand, if one is working single handedly, a great deal of useful information can be gauged from watching the patient walk into the consulting room and take a seat. This can also be the occasion for a little thinking time on the practitioner's part, to decide how best to approach the situation. The client's demeanour can yield clues as to whether they are downcast or walking with difficulty. Whether they respond to a smile and greeting can yield valuable clues as to the likely work needed to establish rapport. A consultation where the practitioner is seen by the client to be caring and attentive need not be a long one. Anecdotes from practitioners and patients describe half-hour consultations which did not yield a sense of satisfaction, whereas warmer, better focused 5-minute ones did so.

To make sense of this, let us draw on another important strand of work in sociology and linguistics that helps to explain how some interactions can imply a great deal more than is actually made explicit. A key idea that is particularly useful is that of 'indexicality', which is seen as a 'method' that individuals employ in creating a sense of intersubjective understanding (Garfinkel 1967; Levinson 1983; Boyle 2000). The term is summarized by Leiter in the following way:

Indexicality refers to the conceptual nature of objects and events. That is to say, without a supplied context, objects and events have equivocal or multiple meanings. The indexical property of talk is the fact that people routinely do not state the intended meaning of the expressions they use. The expressions are vague and equivocal, lending themselves to several meanings. The sense or meaning of these expressions cannot be decided unless a context is supplied. That context consists of such particulars as who the speaker is (his biography), his current purpose and intent, the setting in which the remarks are made, or the actual or potential relationship between speaker and hearer.

(1980: 107)

Within the ethnomethodological tradition, indexicality is not something that individuals find in their environment, and that it is not quite the same as 'world knowledge', 'context-sensitivity', or 'situation'. The kind of context is something that the individuals construct between themselves so as to establish the meaning of what is being said. This kind of construction can proceed very rapidly. Garfinkel (1967: 25–8) claimed that 'for the purpose of *conducting their everyday affairs* persons refuse to permit each other to understand "what they are really talking about" ', because often it is too tiring, time consuming and difficult. Indexicality allows utterances to represent considerably more than is said and thereby makes mundane conversation possible.

Some fragments of this process are disclosed in studies of other service industry groups. In Sharma and Black's (2001) account of the work of 'beauty therapists' there is considerably more than merely offering services such as hairdressing and manicures. The 'pampering' of the client – the morale boosting 'treat'– is delivered in the context of attentiveness to that client's individual needs and circumstances:

When a client comes in you'll say, 'Oh, how did your son's wedding go, how did the party go, did you enjoy that night out, was the film good?' And I think that makes them feel … interesting. Because we all want to feel that as well, we want to feel loved and interesting. And I think [beauty therapists] do that.

(p. 919)

Thus, in a few brief exchanges with a client there is the implication of interest and an implication that the client lives a sufficiently interesting life to be the subject of curiosity. Indeed, the concepts alluded to and the terms deployed, such as wedding, party and the idea of going out to a film are rich with implications of sociability and bonhomie. The interactants do not have to explain what a 'wedding' or 'film' are, nor that the experience might generally be construed as an occasion for enjoyment. Instead the practitioner is able to deploy them to connote a positive experience. This relies upon judgments and values which are 'naturalized' and socially shared, being, as Bourdieu might say, 'transmitted in and through practice'. Indeed one can see the process of using allusive terms which are rich with indexical possibilities as being fundamental to creating space within a relatively condensed encounter. Bourdieu (1980) recognized that the resources or social capital that are inherent in certain social relationships, and the ability to deploy particular symbols or other cultural traits –

'symbolic and cultural capital' – are also an important aspect of the field of power in any society, and from our point of view, they are important inasmuch as they play a part in the reproduction of relationships between practitioners and clients.

In making sense of the indexicality of a statement, a good deal of everyday, commonsensical and arguably shared knowledge is involved. This is also true for researchers seeking to understand what is going on. Garfinkel (1967: 77) intimated that when researchers are engaged in an investigation, they can only make sense of the phenomena under study by drawing on background cultural knowledge. People making sense tend to embed the particular instance in front of them in their 'pre-supposed knowledge of social structures', attending to the sequence of action which unfolds, and waiting for patterns to emerge, even in the shortest of exchanges. The phenomena or patterns that observers see remind them of what has gone before, and the reflexive relationship between past and present helps to contextualize what is happening now, and enables us to predict the future development of a course of action or 'logic of practice'. As Bourdieu describes it, for researchers to understand the logic of practice of a research participant, they must be able to situate themselves imagina-tively 'in the place the interviewee occupies in the social space in order to understand them as *necessarily what they are*' (1996: 22, emphasis in original), in their 'distinctive necessity' (p. 24), such that each participant's 'world-vision becomes self-evident, necessary, *taken for granted*' (emphasis in original).

This reliance on shared meanings can enable relatively brief fragments of con-versation to mean a great deal and can, if used judiciously, enable practitioners and clients to conjointly create 'time tardises' in relatively brief clinical encounters.

The terms we use, then, are rich with culturally encoded shared meanings. Sometimes the indexicality of the concepts used and their connotations create opportunities for upset too. Indexicality is clearly not always about embellishing the encounter with positive connotations or establishing rapport. As we saw in the section about bad news, diagnostic terms sometimes carry an almost unbearable weight for the recipient. To illustrate this, we will provide a quotation from a semi-autobiographical research study by Sara Green who discusses the experience of having a child with disabilities:

> The diagnosing physician is almost universally seen by parents as impossibly distant from their emotional reality (Featherstone 1980; Green and Murton 1996; Quine and Rutter 1994). In our case, Amanda's 'life sentence' was pronounced by a paediatric neurologist we had never seen before in an office visit lasting less than 20 minutes and punctuated by several routine telephone calls and messages regarding other patients. The life stories we had imagined for ourselves and our daughter were obliterated with a few simple words delivered without any sign of emotion: 'has anyone told you that your child has cerebral palsy? No, well that's what she has'. We were assured that 'at least she's not retarded – her head's the right size', and sent on our way armed with a one-page handout of textbook medical definitions – most of which had nothing to do with cerebral palsy and none of which had anything to do with our pain.

(2001: 804–5)

This story, incorporated into an academic account of the care process, highlights a number of factors. Not only do we have the usually unhappy account of being told a 'bad news' diagnosis, but a number of aspects suggest even less propitious circumstances. 'Has anyone told you' alludes to the fragmented nature of the care, and the possibility that the health professionals have known for a while but merely not disclosed the diagnosis. The supplementary information 'at least she's not retarded' and information sheet are felt to have increased rather than decreased the burden, and hint ominously at more dire things to come. The indexicality of the diagnostic terms and the circumstances surrounding the disclosure then spread out beyond the encounter to affect the lives of those concerned over and above coping with the child's physical disabilities.

Sometimes, the unpicking of these negative indexicalities takes a good deal longer than it does to start them off in the first place. One of Green's informants describes a more hopeful encounter with a clinician, some time after receiving the initial diagnosis.

> To this day, I thank this one doctor in the hospital because ... he pulled me aside and he said: 'you know you're hearing a lot of negative ... I want to show you another case . . .' He showed me this one little boy that he had ... delivered eight or nine years before. He had a picture of the kid's brain scan and it was very similar to (hers) ... He said: 'Just get involved as soon as you can with therapy and preventative type things and you'd be surprised. Don't ever let anyone tell you that that child can't do anything. You just bring her home and treat her as normal as possible and don't protect her. Don't baby her. Let her do the best she can do because that's the best you can do for her as a parent'. Then he showed me a picture of this boy when he was eight or nine years old and he was playing baseball and I was like: 'Oh, yes!!'
> (p. 809)

The process of picking apart the negative connotations of diagnostic labels applied by health care professionals may require concentrated, prolonged and complex work. However, this illustrates the same kinds of processes that we have been discussing throughout this chapter. The idea that deceptively ordinary things – pictures of children playing ball games, for example – can be fundamental to achieving good communication in health care contexts is central to the notion of brief communication. While events like these look ordinary, they are filled with interactive work which is much more subtle and complex, and may leave lasting positive impressions.

Conclusion: the possibilities for brief communication

In this chapter therefore we have endeavoured to address a kind of communication suited to the brief encounters of contemporary health care in developed nations. Bourdieu et al. argue that 'narratives about the most "personal" difficulties, the apparently most strictly subjective tensions and contradictions, frequently articulate the deepest structures of the social world and their contradictions' (1993: 511). Thus, the sense a client gains from a health care encounter that they are being listened to, respected or taken seriously and that their fate matters to the health care professional is understandable within a matrix that incorporates the health care system and the culture within which they are embedded as a whole. Moreover, these subjective feelings can be understood once we begin to apply some insights from linguistics, sociology, social psychology and anthropology. These disciplines give us some conceptual and practical tools to begin to enhance the positive processes which we have detected, all of which are applicable to conversations between clients and practitioners lasting five minutes or less. Understanding the value of phatic communication, grasping the significance of emotion work or sentimental work and appreciating how language can mean very much more to interactants than the dictionary definition of the words via the concept of indexicality – these can all contribute to practitioners' ability to communicate effectively with clients.

It is also apparent that much of what is effective in brief communicative encounters is the kind of talk which has typically slipped beneath the radar of health care professionals and educators. It might be described as the 'small talk' (Coupland 2000; McCarthy 2003). Sometimes it is difficult to know exactly where to place the distinction between the relational and the transactional aspects of a conversational exchange in institutional settings (Candlin 2000: xv). Indeed, in some highly condensed encounters there may be a variety of informational and phatic aspects to a single utterance. Erving Goffman was reported to say: 'what talkers undertake to do is not to provide information to a recipient but to present dramas to an audience. Indeed, it seems that we spend most of our time not engaged in giving information but in giving shows' (cited in James 2000: 183). Our theorizing around brief communication has led to the development of a new framework for communication in health care, the Brief, Ordinary and Effective (BOE) model (Crawford et al 2006), which informed the Department of Health's recent guidelines on best practice in mental health nursing (Department of Health 2006).

Alvin Toffler's vision was that large scale mass manufacturing would dwindle and instead a kind of 'recipient tailoring' would come to predominate in industrial production. In a sense the vision of brief communication and its potential that we have attempted to outline here adheres to a similar vision. Perhaps the brevity of so many health care encounters means that increasingly clinicians will have to move away from the large scale 'people processing' (Prottas 1979) and towards a communicative health regimen where participants are attended to individually. Despite their fleeting and transient quality, it may be that the aspects of brief communication we have outlined here can play an increasing role in health care as the brief encounter is elaborated into the art form it should surely be in tomorrow's health services.

References

Bolton, S.C. (2001) Changing faces: nurses as emotional jugglers, *Sociology of Health and Illness*, 23(1): 85–100.

Bosk, C. (1979) *Forgive and Remember: Managing Medical Failure*. Chicago: University of Chicago Press.

Bou-Franch, P. and Garces-Conejos, P. (2003) Teaching linguistic politeness: a methodological proposal, *International Review of Applied Linguistics*, 22: 1–22.

Bourdieu, P. (1980) *The Logic of Practice*. Cambridge: Polity Press.

Bourdieu, P. (1996) Understanding (translated by B. Fowler), *Theory, Culture, and Society: Explorations in Critical Social Science*, 13(2): 17–37.

Bourdieu, P., Accardo, A., Balazs, G., Beaud, S. et al. (1993) *The Weight of the World: Social Suffering in Contemporary Society* (translated by P.P. Ferguson et al.). Stanford, CA: Stanford University Press.

Boyle, R. (2000) 'You've worked with Elizabeth Taylor': phatic functions and implicit compliments, *Applied Linguistics*, 21(1): 26–46.

Brotheridge, C.M. and Lee, R. (2003) Development and validation of the Emotional Labor Scale, *Journal of Occupational and Organizational Psychology*, 76: 365–79.

Brown, B., Nolan, P., Crawford, P. and Lewis, A. (1996) Interaction, language and the narrative turn in psychology and psychiatry, *Social Science and Medicine*, 43(11): 1569–78.

Brown, P. and Levinson, S. (1987) *Politeness: Some Universals in Language Usage*. Cambridge: Cambridge University Press.

Burnard, P. (2003) Ordinary chat and therapeutic conversation: phatic communication and mental health nursing, *Journal of Psychiatric and Mental Health Nursing*, 10: 678–82.

Candlin, C. (2000) General editor's preface, in J. Coupland (ed.) *Small Talk*. London: Longman.

Carter, R. (2004) *Language and Creativity: The Art of Common Talk*. London: Routledge.

Christakis, D.A. and Feudtner, C. (1997) Temporary Matters, *Journal of the American Medical Association*, 278: 739–43.

Coupland, J. (ed.) (2000) *Small Talk*. London: Longman.

Coupland, J., Coupland, N. and Robinson, J.D. (1992) 'How are you?' Negotiating phatic communication, *Language in Society*, 21: 207–30.

Crawford, P., Brown, B. and Bonham, P. (2006) *Communication in Clinical Settings*. Cheltenham: Nelson Thornes.

Department of Health (2006) *Best practice competencies and capabilities for pre-registration mental health nurses in England. The Chief Nursing Officer's review of mental health nursing*. London: The Stationery Office.

Featherstone, H. (1980) *A Difference in the Family: Living with a Disabled Child*. New York: Basic Books.

Fox, S. (1990) The ethnography of humour and the problem of social reality, *Sociology*, 24: 431–46.

Garfinkel, H. (1967) *Studies in Ethnomethodology*. Englewood Cliffs, NJ: Prentice Hall.

Global Commission on International Migration (2004) *Global Migration Perspectives: Migrants, Labour Markets and Integration in Europe: a Comparative Analysis*. Geneva: Global Commission on International Migration.

Goffman, E. (1955) On face-work: an analysis of ritual elements in social interaction, *Psychiatry: Journal for the Study of Interpersonal Processes*, 18: 213–31.

Goffman, E. (1967) *Interaction Rituals: Essays in Face-to-face Behaviour*. Chicago: Aldine.

Green, J. and Murton, F. (1996) Diagnoses of Duchenne muscular dystrophy: parents' experiences and satisfaction, *Child: Care, Health and Development*, 22: 13–28.

Green, S.E. (2001) 'Oh, those therapists will become your best friends': maternal satisfaction with clinics providing physical, occupational and speech therapy services to children with disabilities, *Sociology of Health and Illness*, 23(6): 798–828.

Hochschild, A. (1983) *The Managed Heart: Commercialization of Human Feeling*. Berkeley, CA: University of California Press.

Irvine-Doran, D., Sidani, S., Keatings, M. and Doige, D. (2002) An empirical test of the Nursing Role Effectiveness Model, *Journal of Advanced Nursing*, 38(1): 29–39.

James, D. (2000) *Dona Maria's Story: Life History, Memory, and Political Identity*. Chapel Hill, NC: Duke University Press.

Jefferson, G. (1984) On the organization of laughter in talk about troubles, in J.M. Atkinson and J. Heritage (eds) *Structures of Social Action: Studies in Conversation Analysis*. Cambridge: Cambridge University Press.

Jefferson, G., Sacks, H. and Schegloff, E. (1987) Notes on laughter in the pursuit of intimacy, in G. Button and J.R.E. Lee (eds) *Talk and Social Organization*. Clevedon: Multilingual Matters.

Kasper, G. (1992) Pragmatic transfer, *Second Language Research*, 8: 203–31.

Lakoff, R.T. (1989) The limits of politeness: therapeutic and courtroom discourse, *Multilingua*, 8: 101–29.

Laver, J.D.M.H. (1975) Communicative functions of phatic communion, in A. Kendon, R.M. Harris and M.R. Key (eds) *The Organization of Behavior in Face-to-face Interaction*. The Hague: Mouton.

Laver, J.D.M.H. (1981) Linguistic routines and politeness in greeting and parting, in F. Coulmas (ed.) *Conversational Routine: Explorations in Standardized Communication Situations and Prepatterned Speech*. The Hague: Mouton.

Leiter, K. (1980) *A Primer on Ethnomethodology*. Oxford: Oxford University Press.

Levinson, S.C. (1983) *Pragmatics*. Cambridge: Cambridge University Press.

McCarthy, M.J. (2003) Talking back: 'small' interactional response tokens in everyday conversation, in J. Coupland (ed.) *Research on Language and Social Interaction* (special issue on 'small talk'), 36(1): 33–63.

McColl, A., Smith, H., White, P. and Field, J. (1998) General practitioners' perceptions of the route to evidence-based medicine: a questionnaire survey, *British Medical Journal*, 316: 361–5.

McCoy, L. (2005) HIV-positive patients and the doctor–patient relationship: perspectives from the margins, *Qualitative Health Research*, 15(6): 791–806.

Malinowski, B. (1922) *Argonauts of the Western Pacific: An Account of Native Enterprise and Adventure in the Archipelago of Melanesian New Guinea*. London: Routledge.

Mann, S. and Cowburn, J. (2005) Emotional labour and stress within mental health nursing, *Journal of Psychiatric and Mental Health Nursing*, 12: 154–62.

NHS Direct (2006) *Walk in Centres*. Available at http://www.nhsdirect.nhs.uk/en.aspx?articleID=418 (accessed 18 March 2006)

O'Brien, M. (1994) The managed heart revisited: health and social control, *Sociological Review*, 42: 393–413.

Phillips, S. (1996) Labouring the emotions: expanding the remit of nursing work? *Journal of Advanced Nursing*, 24: 139–43.

Prottas, J.M. (1979) *People-processing*. Lexington, MA: Lexington Books.

Quine, L. and Rutter, D.R. (1994) First diagnosis of severe mental and physical disability: a study of doctor–parent communication, *Journal of Child Psychology and Psychiatry*, 35: 1273–87.

Sacks, H., Schegloff, E.A. and Jefferson, G. (1974) A simplest systematics for the organization of turn-taking for conversation, *Language*, 50: 696–735.

Scollon, R. and Scollon, S.W. (1995) *Intercultural Communication: A Discourse Approach*. Cambridge, MA: Blackwell.

Serrant-Green, L. (2005) Breaking traditions: sexual health and ethnicity in nursing research: a literature review, *Journal of Advanced Nursing*, 51(5): 511–19.

Sharma, U. and Black, P. (2001) Look good, feel better: beauty therapy as emotional labour, *Sociology*, 35(4): 913–31.

Shattrell, M. (2004) Nurse–patient interaction: a review of the literature, *Journal of Clinical Nursing*, 13: 714–22.

Staden, H. (1998) Alertness to the needs of others: a study of the emotional labour of caring, *Journal of Advanced Nursing*, 27: 147–56.

Strauss, A., Fagerhaugh, S., Suczek, B. and Wiener, C. (1982) Sentimental work in the technologized hospital, *Sociology of Health and Illness*, 4: 255–78.

Sudnow, D. (1967) *Passing On*. Englewood Cliffs, NJ: Prentice Hall.

Thomas, J. (1983) Cross-cultural pragmatic failure, *Applied Linguistics*, 4: 91–112.

Toffler, A. (1980) *The Third Wave*. New York: William Morrow and Co.

Tomlin, Z., Humphrey, C. and Rogers, S. (1999) General practitioners' perceptions of effective health care, *British Medical Journal*, 318: 1532–5.

Young, J.M. and Ward, J.E. (2001) Evidence-based medicine in general practice: beliefs and barriers among Australian GPs, *Journal of Evaluation in Clinical Practice*, 7(2): 201–10.

11 Conclusion

This final chapter will conclude our consideration of communication in relation to evidence-based health care. It is a difficult task to simply summarize what has been learned so far concerning the study and teaching of communication in health care and what we know about the methodology for evaluating effective communication strategies and communication teaching styles. In many cases, the findings that research has yielded seem frustratingly banal, concerning the need to be polite to patients, look at them rather than one's notes or computer screen, use terms they can understand, use open rather than closed questions and so on.

Maybe this isn't merely stating the obvious though. Perhaps what we are facing when clients or patients complain about the kinds of communicative experiences they have is not just a failure of communication. Maybe it tells us something fundamental about how health care is managed and delivered. Practitioners are faced with increasing pressures to be especially careful in compiling notes, entering the correct information into databases and attending to their documentation. Indeed, anecdotal evidence from clinically based colleagues is yielding stories about how failure to complete the electronic records is a disciplinary offence in some parts of the UK. Whether this will make records any more complete or accurate is a debatable point. It will certainly involve new layers of management and bureaucracy to administer and much time will be spent in meetings and tribunals. In the light of these movements in health care itself it is little wonder that clinicians appear more interested in the electronic or paper records than they are in their patients. Little wonder also that research and communications skills training has to remind them that the person in the bed, or opposite them in the consulting room, needs a little attention too.

It is customary also to offer, amidst one's conclusions, suggestions for further research and exploration based on some of the recent developments in the field. This would perhaps be to overestimate the power of a single book to influence the agenda. The study of health care language proceeds apace, and its future direction is an emergent property which will surely have little to do with our admonishments. Nevertheless it is tempting to step up onto the soapbox afforded by the concluding chapter and the experience of relief at having got this far in the face of pressing deadlines.

As the reader will have noticed by now, we are not uncritical of notions of evidence-based practice itself. As it is currently formulated, it is not necessarily geared to the evaluation and dissemination of communicative practice for it is still dominated by notions of research which privilege the randomized controlled clinical trial. The authors, and some health care professionals too, believe that there are important, health-promoting interpersonal qualities in communication which have yet to be captured by conventional modes of evidence-based practice. Furthermore, evidence-based practice is often seen by health professionals as a bugbear rather than an asset, a process which increases surveillance, interventionist management styles and paperwork at the expense of patient care.

One of the major suggestions we would make having proceeded through the fields of enquiry covered in this volume is that we need to broaden the study of health care communication to include the contexts and cultures that surround the consultation or advice-giving episode. It is here that the practical meaning of the communicative episode can best be understood. Perhaps apparent failures in communication in the consulting room, at the bedside or in the community are traceable not to deficits in skills and knowledge but to differences in culture, frameworks of understanding, lifestyles and priorities. People are enacting socially embedded identities and appreciating this will open up analytic possibilities that are missed with static conceptions of identity knowledge and skill. Many theories, especially those with a social-psychological focus, tend to essentialize the people in a clinical encounter and assume the unity of an inner self.

There are alternatives to this position. As Bamberg (2004: 6) describes it, selves and identities are 'projects . . . constantly under revision . . . tested out by interactants'. As Riessman (2003) adds, constructing 'who I am' is an ongoing activity with a context-specific range and is a practical project of everyday life (see also Holstein and Gubrium 2002).

This is not to say that a person in a health care context has freedom to construct an identity in a voluntaristic, 'pic'n'mix' manner. The sheer obdurate burden of illness often makes freedom seem like a very distant memory indeed. Yet even in the face of this, people actively construct and revise the social self. At the very least, says Riessman (2003), narrators control the terms of storytelling, they occupy 'privileged positions in story worlds of their own creation' (Patterson 2002: 2). Consequently, if we conceptualize these accounts as performances, narratives of the kind we dealt with in Chapter 4 can be seen as courses of action in their own right, as intentional projects (Skultans 2000: 9). The implication for the study of health care communication is that these stories are a whole lot more than accounts of alleged events that happened in the past. They are a performance that constructs identity in the present. Therefore our analytic focus should shift from 'the told' – the events to which language refers – to include 'the telling' (Mishler 1995; Riessman 2003).

Stories about feeling ill, about the progress of treatment, family difficulties or even stories about how little you know are all kinds of performances enacted between culturally astute members of a particular community. Williams (1999: 247) argues that 'illness has become something of a trope upon which to hang all kinds of musings about the meaning of damaged bodies and damaged lives'. Stories have a potential healing function, in that they provide a form to link the past, present, and an imagined future. In addition, as we tell stories about our own health or how we can improve other people's, identity work is being accomplished through these culturally meaningful performances. In this view, which owes as much to Judith Butler or Erving Goffman as it does to Pierre Bourdieu, the human condition is seen as enacting, performing and displaying, making ourselves intelligible against a particular cultural background using shared discursive tools.

Partly, these shared discursive tools involve the deposits left in the culture by social scientists themselves. As Bell (2000: 186) writes, 'understanding the experience of illness involves more than "simply" the experiences of others; it also involves the experiences of sociologists attempting to understand the experiences of others'. The study of health care communication leaves traces that change the contexts and opportunities for people to make sense of and tell stories about their distress.

Certainly, it is by assiduous, meticulous attention to the fine-grained texture of interaction in health care contexts that evidence-based communication can be realized as a technique that can genuinely enhance the practice of skilled caring practitioners and help to ensure that their expertise is available to train the next generation of helping professionals. However, there is more to a genuinely evidence-based communication than this. Our regular return to the work of Pierre Bourdieu throughout this volume has, we hope, highlighted the necessity of seeing the cultural context and the habitus that is being acted out by the participants in health care as they interact. It involves seeing the kinds of cultural functions and meanings that people's stories have in their homes, families and communities. Appearing to soldier on bravely in the face of arthritis, having a family life devoted to the care of others, or being a sole wage earner in a competitive and demanding environment may all have a bearing on the kinds of health care communication that are entered into. It is by attending to the ideas of context and culture, by addressing what has variously been called culture, 'habitus', pragmatics and 'indexicality' over the course of this volume, that we can build a genuinely 'evidence-based' and practice relevant strategy for communication in health care.

References

Bamberg, M. (2004) 'We are young, responsible, and male', *Human Development*, 47(6): 331–53.

Bell, S.E. (2000) 'Experiencing illness in/and narrative', in C.E. Bird, P. Conrad and A.M. Fremont (eds) *Handbook of Medical Sociology*, 5th edn. Upper Saddle River, NJ: Prentice Hall.

Holstein, J.A. and Gubrium, J.F. (2002) *The Self We Live By: Narrative Identity in a Postmodern World*. New York: Oxford University Press.

Mishler, E.G. (1995) Models of narrative analysis: a typology, *Journal of Narrative and Life History*, 5(2): 87–123.

Patterson, W. (ed.) (2002) *Strategic Narrative: New Perspectives on the Power of Personal and Cultural Storytelling*. Lanham, MD: Lexington Books.

Riessman, C.K. (2003) Performing identities in illness narrative: masculinity and multiple sclerosis, *Qualitative Research*, 3(1): 5–33.

Skultans, V. (2000): Narrative, illness and the body (editorial), *Anthropology and Medicine*, 7(1): 5–13.

Williams, G. (1999) Bodies on a battlefield: the dialectics of disability (review article), *Sociology of Health and Illness*, 21(2): 242–52.

Index

PATIENT PARTICIPATION IN HEALTH CARE CONSULTATIONS

**Sarah Collins, Nicky Britten, Johanna Ruusuvuori
and Andrew Thompson**

- How does patient participation work in practice?
- What does it look like when it happens?
- Why is it being promoted?
- How can it be researched, and how can it be taught?

This book addresses all these questions with each chapter developing a particular angle. The book provides answers by exploring interconnections between theory, research and practice, and by drawing on different disciplinary perspectives in the health and social sciences. It invites comparisons between different health care settings and combines patient, professional and academic perspectives.

Contributors: *Sarah Collins, Nicky Britten, Carol Bugge, John Chatwin, Rowena Field, Joseph Gafaranga, Aled Jones, Pirjo Lindfors, Anssi Perakyla, Johanna Ruusuvuori, Fiona Stevenson, Andrew Thompson, Ian Watt.*

Contents: *Part I - Setting the scene: debates on patient participation, and methods for studying it - Introduction - Putting participation into words: a conceptualisation - Methods for studying patient participation - The meaning of patient involvement and participation: a taxonomy - Part II - Participation in practice - What's a good consultation and what's a bad one? The patient perspective - Reflections on the concept of participation in general practice in health care consultations - What is patient participation? Comparing patient participation in three different health care settings - A feeling of equality: some interactional features of a homoeopathic therapeutic encounter - Nursing assessments and other tasks: some constraints on participation in interaction between patients and nurses - Part III - A conceptual overview of participation - Components of participation: a methodological framework - An integrative approach to patient involvement in consultations: components, levels, and contexts - Conclusions: making links between research, policy, education and practice.*

224pp   0 335 21964 0 Paperback   0 335 21965 9 Hardback

HEALTH COMMUNICATION: THEORY AND PRACTICE

Dianne Berry

- Why is effective communication important in health, and what does this involve?
- What issues arise when communicating with particular populations, or in difficult circumstances?
- How can the communication skills of health professionals be improved?

Effective health communication is now recognised to be a critical aspect of healthcare at both the individual and wider public level. Good communication is associated with positive health outcomes, whereas poor communication is associated with a number of negative outcomes. This book assesses current research and practice in the area and provides some practical guidance for those involved in communicating health information. It draws on material from several disciplines, including health, medicine, psychology, sociology, linguistics, pharmacy, statistics, and business and management.

The book examines:

- The importance of effective communication in health
- Basic concepts and processes in communication
- Communication theories and models
- Communicating with particular groups and in difficult circumstances
- Ethical issues
- Communicating with the wider public and health promotion
- Communication skills training

Health Communication is key reading for students and researchers who need to understand the factors that contribute to effective communication in health, as well as for health professionals who need to communicate effectively with patients and others. It provides a thorough and up to date, evidence-based overview of this important topic, examining the theoretical and practical aspects of health communication for those whose work involves communication with patients, relatives and other carers.

Contents: *Preface - Introduction to Health Communication - Basic Forms of Communication – Underlying Theories and Models - Communication between Patients and Health Professionals - Communicating with Particular Populations in Healthcare - Communication of Difficult Information and in Difficult Circumstances - Health Promotion and Communication with the Wider Public - Communication Skills Training – References – Index.*

152pp   0 335 21870 9 Paperback   0 335 21871 7 Hardback

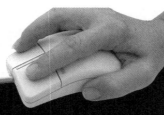